AL

CW00548317

Discover How to Cleanse Your Body and Improve
Your Life

(How to Induce Your Body's Natural Detox
Process for Weight Loss)

Addie Houston

Published by Tomas Edwards

© **Addie Houston**

All Rights Reserved

Autophagy Book: Discover How to Cleanse Your Body and Improve Your Life (How to Induce Your Body's Natural Detox Process for Weight Loss)

ISBN 978-1-989744-93-2

Legal & Disclaimer

The information contained in this book is not designed to replace or take the place of any form of medicine or professional medical advice. The information in this book has been provided for educational and entertainment purposes only.

The information contained in this book has been compiled from sources deemed reliable, and it is accurate to the best of the Author's knowledge; however, the Author cannot guarantee its accuracy and validity and cannot be held liable for any errors or omissions. Changes are periodically made to this book. You must consult your doctor or get professional medical advice before using any of the

Table of Contents

Introduction To The Intermittent Fasting

The Concept behind the Intermittent Fasting

We are so fortunate to be alive at this time when we have an abundant supply of food. We're fortunate to be living at the time that we can choose to eat wherever and whatever we like. We are so fortunate to be living in this modern era of surplus food and abundance.

Even though we're living in the modern era of food abundance, our body still functions like it did when our ancestors were living in caves, gathering their food and hunting for their foods. Food was very scarce in the time of our ancestors, so their bodies had to create mechanisms to cope with the food scarcity that loomed at that time. Their bodies had to come up with clear waking times and clear sleeping times for them. They ate when they were awake and fasted while they were sleeping.

However, even though our body still functions like it did during the time of our ancestors, technology is changing that for us. We now have an abundance of food and we are definitely sleeping less than we are supposed to do. Hence, we are now eating more food over a longer period of the day than our bodies are designed for. We are constantly overeating. Our ancestors did not do so.

That's why we have more cases of diabetes, overweight, sugar cravings, slow metabolism and a host of other issues more than what our forefathers had.

Thus, the idea of intermittent fasting is to shrink our eating window to be more inclined with the original natural design of the body.

Keep in mind that the intermittent fasting is not against the notion that we have to keep our metabolism stable by having snacks throughout the day or keep a bag of nuts nearby to have more intakes of protein and fiber in the body.

The intermittent fasting is designed to find a middle ground for your body. It's designed to give your body a break from too much food so that your body doesn't spend too much energy on trying to digest and eliminate the foods that you're consuming.

The energy that our bodies spend today in trying to digest and expel foods from our digestive system can be used for repairing and making the body to recover.

The intermittent fasting is mostly concerned with increasing the sleeping hours of your day and reducing the waking hours of your day. Because when you are eating more, you tend to be more awake than when you are fasting.

So intermittent fasting really limits your eating to the most wakening hours of the day so that you are more active during those periods. Then it limits the body's activities during the night time and the morning times so that it can really work on rebuilding the body's worn-out tissue.

How to succeed on the intermittent fasting

The intermittent fasting still works and will continue to work well for decades. If you've never tried the intermittent fasting before, then, it's really hard to make the cold switch to go from an eating state to a fasting state. What this implies is that intermittent fasting can sometimes be extremely tough especially at the beginning.

For the intermittent fasting to be a success for you, you need to look at your eating pattern before you decide that you are only going to stop eating by 7pm and resume eating again by 9 pm.

So look at your current pattern of eating right now. If you are still currently having some snacks by 11pm, then it'll be extremely difficult for you to stop doing that and start having your last meal at 7pm, what you want to do is to start shifting your last eating meal hour by one hour every single week. So if your last meal was 11pm before, you can decide to bring it down to 10pm this week, and then next week reduce it to 9pm and then 8pm, the week that follows that until you start eating your last meal by 7pm.

Also, you need to start checking how you're reacting to the fasting. Check the quality of your sleep as you are undergoing the fasting. Check the number of your hunger levels and your mood fluctuations throughout your fasting.

You can do all that by getting an old school spiral notebook and a pen and taking a lot of notes about how your body feels so that you can know the patterns of your body. It's not going to be possible to remember the things that you eat every single day or the number of hours that you're sleeping every day, that's why keeping a notebook by your side to take notes is going to be super beneficial to you.

You can also use a wearable digital fitness tracker to track your body patterns. One of the core keys to having successful intermittent fasting is to see yourself as an experiment and a work in progress. Intermittent fasting doesn't really stand on its own.

It's something that you can combine with a host of other healthy things so that you can see the benefits of your fasting. If you want to see the most benefits from your intermittent fasting, then you have to start to eat healthy foods, cut all processed sugar and become very active.

You have to be ready to start living a healthy lifestyle if you want to get the most benefits of your fasting. You can't just wake up one morning in your unhealthy lifestyle and decide that you're going to start limiting the hours that you're eating. You have to really plan ahead to fully get the benefits of the fasting.

How to get the full benefits of the intermittent fasting

The real benefits of the intermittent fasting in your body will be determined by these three glands; your thyroid, adrenaline glands and the Hyperthalamus and the communication between the thyroid, the hypertalus, and the adrenaline glands. Those three things also play a huge role in the metabolism in our body.

If any of these three glands are not working well, then you are not really going to see the effect of the intermittent fasting in your life. The hypothalamus is the gland that controls the temperature of the body system.

As we age, we tend to shy away from doing resistant exercises because we don't want to hurt our body, or look stupid.

Therefore, we just go back to doing little or no exercise at all. So to boost our metabolism, we need to start doing resistant exercises that will stimulate the hypothalamus and will regulate body temperature. Doing resistant training will help to fire your body from the inside, which in turn will boost up the metabolism.

What we'll talk about in this book

In this book, we'll go through an overview of the intermittent fasting, why you should do it. We'll talk about what intermittent fasting is and why you shouldn't overthink it. We'll talk about the basic benefits.

We'll concentrate so many notes on the benefits of intermittent fasting because if you're reading this book, you're probably already interested in the intermittent fasting because you know someone that had crazy benefits with it. We will talk about the physical benefits like fat loss and some muscle gain.

We will talk about cellular and rejuvenation benefits also known as metabolism autophagy. So in detail, we'll be talking about how to start a fast, what you should do before fasting.

Then we will talk about how long you should fast, how much time you should spend on your fasting periods. Then we will talk about what you can and cannot consume during your fasting period.

You will know if you should consume coffee or tea while fasting. Next, we will talk about how to break a fast. Then we will talk about whether you should actually workout during your fasting, or better still if you should even workout at all. We will talk about the different types of fasting. There's intermittent fasting. There's the liquid fasting. There is prolonged fasting. There are different kinds of fasting, you just have to know the one that is right for you.

Then we talk about the fasting process for men and women, some slight differences that you have to pay attention to for you to make your fasting experience better. Then we will talk about the common concerns of fasting.

You have to read to the end of the book to get this aspect. The section that will talk about the common concerns of fasting will connect all the dots of everything in the book and will help you get rid of any confusion that you are currently having.

We will talk about the muscle loss concerns and also the fibroid just in case you're wondering if intermittent fasting will slow down your metabolism. We will talk about when you should take your supplements.

You will know if you should take the supplements during your supplement period or when you are eating. We will talk about alcohol consumption, whether the alcohol will break your fast or not.

Chapter 1: What Is Autophagy?

AUTOPHAGY IS JUST one of a number of cellular processes utilized by the human body to help it achieve equilibrium. This equilibrium is what allows the human body to be the well-oiled machine that it is: an instrument that is capable of engaging in a wide variety of cellular processes and meet the basic demands for life. Indeed, it is easy to take for granted all that the human body does and how well it does it. The human body is able to manage several different complex organ systems, breakdown nutrients to meet energy and molecular requirements, turn waste products into molecules that can be removed from the body, just to name a few of the major things the human body is able to do.

Our body would not be able to do all this if it was burdened with parts that were damaged or not functioning at all. Just as companies shift employees to different roles or terminate them if they are no longer able to complete their necessary functions, the human body is also required to engage in this management process. It may seem strange to make the analogy of a human being and a business, but it really is not a stretch. The human body is extremely complex, and it can be argued that the body manages its many tasks even better than most businesses can.

In order to keep itself functioning properly, the human body has to be a little heartless when it comes to removing components that are not needed, damaged, require changed, or are otherwise antithetical to what the body needs. The body accomplishes this turnover of cells through what is known as cell death. Cell death is the general term for the demise of the cell, the basic constituent of life for organisms on Earth, and this process can be carefully triggered and managed by the body through complex signaling pathways.

Cell death is often used by people to refer to the process by which the body turns over cells naturally, although it also encompasses the reality of cells that die due to injury, cancer, or other traumatic means. Cell death is a wider term that includes several categories, but it is convenient to think of cell death in terms of apoptotic and non-apoptotic cell death. Apoptotic cell death refers to the well-known process of apoptosis. Apoptosis is a type of programmed cell death that involves a cell carefully destroying itself in a routine pattern that can be visualized on an electron microscope. Non-apoptotic cell death refers to means of cell-degradation that occur outside of apoptosis.

Introduction to Autophagy

Autophagy is a type of non-apoptotic cell death. This should not give you the impression that autophagy is somehow haphazard or occurs outside of a body plan or program. The body is able to regulate the process of autophagy just as it is able to mitigate other types of cell death, including apoptosis. Autophagy was long a realm of scientific knowledge that was little known to people or confusing. At present, enough is known about autophagy that writers are able to write books about them (like this one), tailored to specific aspects of this process. In this book, autophagy will be discussed from the standpoint of how it can be used to achieve specific health and fitness goals.

Although autophagy occurs in cell death, its implications reach far outside the realm of helping the body maintain normal equilibrium. Because autophagy is mediated by a number of genes that lead to the expression of specific proteins and signaling molecules, autophagy can be the target of drugs or other therapeutic agents. For some of you, the implication of that statement is readily apparent. Autophagy can be utilized to destroy tumors (cancer cells) or sites of infection. Most autophagy genes have been discovered through the study of fungi, and the number of genes that are known is increasingly (currently, about ten autophagy genes are known).

The study of autophagy resulted in the awarding of a Nobel Prize to Yoshinori Ohsumi in 2016. This prize was awarded in part because of information about autophagy genes, which expanded on the original knowledge of lysosomal function that was associated with the coining of the term autophagy in the 1960s. It could be said that the lysosome is the basic unit necessary for autophagy to occur, but in fact, autophagy genes involve a complex signaling process of amino acids and enzymes. This topic will be discussed further in the next chapter.

What is important for you to know by way of an introduction to autophagy is that this process has a number of functions. Although, as stated previously, autophagy occurs in non-apoptotic cell death, it also occurs in other homeostatic processes that do not involve the death of the cell. For example, studies on mice have shown that autophagy is necessary for the maintenance of muscle homeostasis as well as homeostasis of the body as a whole. Homeostasis merely refers to the conditions the body or an organ of the body needs to maintain its normal functions: such as temperature, pH, and the like.

Most studies of autophagy as a natural process (aside from therapeutic uses in cancer and infection) involve knocking out one or more of the known autophagy genes in mice. In other words, scientists block the action of one of these genes thereby preventing the expression of the molecule the gene encodes. This will result in a specific loss of function in these mammals (usual mice), which allows the researchers to make deductions about the purpose of the gene and the overall utility of autophagy in normal body homeostasis.

For example, studies have shown that when a specific autophagy gene is knocked out in mice, these mice experience problems with the metabolism of glucose and endurance during exercise. This particular gene was involved in marking proteins for metabolism. In other words, letting a muscle cell know that a particular protein was ready to be broken down. This is significant for a number of reasons. For one thing, it highlights the basic way that autophagy works – by the cell tagging a molecule for turnover. It also emphasizes that autophagy is critical in the human body outside of the process of cell death.

The body has many uses for autophagy. You will learn about some of this in the e-book you are currently reading. Exercise has been an active area of study, in part because autophagy appears to be very important in maintaining homeostasis within the muscle. Aside from the turnover of proteins, autophagy is also involved in the normal process of contraction of muscle that is necessary to exercise. This subject will be explored further later on in this e-book. Aside from exercise and muscle homeostasis, autophagy is also involved in these other processes:

- Repair of damaged molecules

- Suppression of tumors

- Cell death

- Autophagy of infectious particles (xenophagy)

- Target of infectious agents

- Target of tumor cells

One of the important things to note about autophagy here is that it is not only a normal process within the body, but it is also a target for foreign pathogens or dysfunction processes whose goal is to derail the normal functions of the body. There are viruses that are able to interfere with the normal process of autophagy of infectious particles, like viruses. This allows these infections to resist destruction by the pathway that was designed to remove them. This is also true for tumor cell survival. Tumor cells are able to downregulate autophagy to allow their own survival, while also rendering them ineffective to radiation. Knocking out these genes selectively in tumors can render those targets of normal autophagy as well as targets of therapeutic treatments like chemotherapy or radiation.

Autophagy and Aging

An interesting topic of discussion in the realm of introduction to autophagy is the role that autophagy normally plays in aging. As hinted at above, autophagy is responsible for maintaining homeostasis in a number of ways, including removing damaged cells or particles from the body through a signaling mechanism. Some scientists believe that as the body gets older, it becomes less efficient at autophagy and therefore there is an accumulation of molecules and cells that would otherwise be removed by autophagy.

The implication here is that making the body more efficient at autophagy or stimulating it, in general, can actually improve longevity. Of course, the goal would not be to stimulate healthy cells or particles in the body to be destroyed through this signaling pathway. The human body (and the bodies of other animals) appears to be pretty good at tagging cells and particles that should be destroyed and leaving the normal ones alone. The idea is to enable this process, to encourage it, so that these damaged cells and particles do not linger and lead to aging.

The overall gestalt here is that the human body becomes less efficient with homeostasis as one gets older. If you can find ways to improve your body's homeostasis, its equilibrium, then you are not only improving your overall health picture but potentially increasing your lifespan. In this e-book, you will see that it is not difficult to push your body in the right way when it comes to this homeostatic picture. You do not need to target genes with medication to do your part (although this can be useful when it comes to cancer treatment or infection). Something as simple as eating the right foods or timing of meals can stimulate homeostasis.

Types of Autophagy

In this chapter, we have introduced you to some of the science behind the process of self-degradation known as autophagy. The goal here has been to allow you to understand the subject enough that the rest of the chapters are more easily digestible when you get to them later. Much more of the science behind autophagy will be addressed in chapter two when we describe precisely how autophagy works. You know now that autophagy works using lysosomes and signaling molecules that tag molecules or cells for destruction, but what are these signaling proteins and how does the process proceed from Point A to Point B.

Before you learn more about those topics, it is important to understand that there are different types of autophagy. You might have gleamed some of this in the discussion about some of the things that autophagy is able to accomplish outside the realm of cell death in a programmed fashion. Autophagy is clearly able to handle normal molecules in the human body, cells, foreign particles, tissues like muscle. This means that autophagy is able to work in various distinct ways suggesting that there are different mechanisms of this process.

Although autophagy is a complicated subject, for the purposes of discussion, it can be divided into three major types based on the overall mechanism of action. Understanding these types of autophagy does make the picture of the molecular process clearer. Autophagy can be divided into these three primary types.

Macroautophagy: This is sometimes referred to as autophagy. This is the process by which a vesicle surrounded by a double membrane (like the cell itself) is delivered to the lysosome to be destroyed by enzymes contained within that organelle. This is the most basic form of autophagy.

Microautophagy: Microautophagy accomplishes the destruction of particles, but by a different means. Using this mechanism, the lysosome engulfs directly the particle that is intended for destruction rather than passively accepting the vesicle containing the particle. This action is referred to as the invagination of the lysosome, meaning that it is surrounding and accepting the particle inside of itself. This has been shown to be an important process in autophagy that occurs in response to environmental changes.

Chaperone-mediated autophagy: This form of autophagy does not involve a double-membrane vesicle or invagination of the lysosome. Instead, particles are tagged with a molecule known as a chaperone that is recognized by receptors on the surface of the lysosome. Once recognized, these tagged particles (proteins) from the cytoplasm are taken into the cell where they are degraded by the lysosomal enzymes.

Autophagy, therefore, is able to accomplish its basic goals of achieving cell and tissue homeostasis by processes that are at once simple and complex. Autophagy on the macro-level becomes more involved as the specific genes and signaling molecules are researched further. But as you can see from this discussion of autophagy in general and the main types of autophagy, this process essentially depends on the body being able to recognize what needs to be degraded. By understanding how the body accomplishes this recognition, you will be able to encourage natural autophagy and improve your own health and longevity.

Chapter 2: How Autophagy Works

By now, the term autophagy is quite familiar to you. You are also aware of the origin and development, as well as the key benefits of autophagy to your overall health. In this chapter, we will strive to understand how autophagy works in your body.

First, it is essential to note that your cells accumulate a lot of dead organelles over time. They also accumulate damaged proteins as well as oxidized particles. The accumulation of these debris clogs and affects your body's inner workings.

When your body's optimal working conditions are affected by the accumulation of the unwanted debris, your aging process is accelerated substantially. Your risk of getting exposure to diseases such as cancer and other age-related disorders such as dementia is also increased significantly.

Your body then develops a unique way of getting rid of the damaged, diseased, or worn-out cells and cell parts to enable crucial cells such as the brain cells to last for a lifetime. This unique way is what is called autophagy and is critical in empowering your body to naturally defend itself against any invasion by disease-causing pathogens.

How Autophagy Works

For you to understand better how autophagy works in your body, we are going to use two analogies:

Analogy 1: In the first analogy, we are going to take your body as a busy kitchen. After you have made your food, you usually keep your kitchen clean by getting rid of any leftovers and any accumulated dirt. The cleaning helps to maintain your kitchen in pristine conditions and makes it conducive for the next meal preparation. You also recycle any food left for use in the subsequent day. This is how autophagy works in your body. It gets rid of any worn-out cells and accumulated debris. It then regenerates new cells which can work better and defend your body against any disease infections.

Analogy 2: We will use the same kitchen scenario, but because of old age, you can't perform your duties of cleaning the kitchen well. So, after cooking, you leave all the dirt behind. They deposit on the counter, and over time, the toxic waste undergoes food fermentation. This results in nasty smells as the food remnants undergo decomposition. Your kitchen becomes a haven of toxins, pollutants, and germs. This is what happens in your body in the absence of autophagy.

The process of autophagy in your body takes place subconsciously and silently behind the scenes as it goes about its maintenance business. However, the process is put into high gear during the periods of extreme stress. This is the natural way through which your response against stress agents such as famine or infections. Activating autophagy in your body, therefore, results in the slowing of the aging process. It also reduces your body's inflammation rates to boost your immune system.

Explanation of Autophagy Process: The Scientific Way

A recent study conducted by Newcastle University reveals that humans can live longer because of the adaptations in a protein commonly known as p62. P62 helps you to respond better when exposed to any biological stressors. The process of autophagy induces the p62 protein.

The P62 protein activates autophagy to start cleansing once it senses metabolic by-products that cause damage in your body. These by-products are scientifically referred to as reactive oxygen species or ROS. The p62 proteins work by removing all damaged and unwanted parts in your cell, enabling you to be better equipped to fight any biological stress. This process is critical for making you look younger and healthier.

The researchers also established that this process is unique to humans. They used fruit flies to understand the process of autophagy in humans. In their studies, the fruit flies failed to kick start the process of autophagy, so the researches sought an explanation for this failure. It was established that the part of the human p62 protein enables your body to sense ROS.

They then created genetically modified flies using humanized p62 protein. The result was that the humanized flies were able to survive for long periods when exposed to stressful conditions as compared to their peers. They concluded that humans had developed their abilities in sensing stress and inactivating their protective processes such as autophagy to fight diseases and live longer.

Autophagy also works to help in the maintenance of homeostasis in your body. During autophagy, your p62 protein helps maintain homeostasis and vibrant health by enabling the damaged cell parts which have accumulated in your body to be turned into new cell formation.

Ways to Accelerate Autophagy in your Body

There are quite a number of effective ways through which you can expedite the process of autophagy in your body. These are proven methods that you can use to cleanse your cells and reduce your body's inflammation rate to keep your body in pristine condition. However, for the methods to work well, you must trick your body into thinking that it is under immense stress.

Eating a high-fat and low-carb meal

A diet high in fat and low in carbs is referred to as a keto diet or ketonic diet. Studies show a keto diet helps to accelerate your autophagy processes. Once you adopt a keto diet, your body is forced to shift from burning g glucose to burning fats. The method of burning fats or ketones mimics what happens typically when you are in a fasted state, and this helps to trigger the autophagy process.

You can replace the sugar intake with fat for your life to be transformed through the process of autophagy. The ketonic diet also helps you to lose weight and live a healthy life.

Go on a protein fast

Another way to accelerate the process of autophagy in your body is by limiting your daily intake of protein. You can start by capping your protein consumption to about 15 to 25 grams per day. Doing this will enable your body to recycle excess proteins. Recycling of excess proteins enables your body to reduce its inflammation rate. Your body will also cleanse its cells even without losing any muscle loss.

During this time, your body will be consuming its protein and toxins through the process of autophagy.

Practice intermittent fasting

Intermittent fasting is the practice through which you limit the intake of your food for specific periods. Intermittent fasting has been shown to accelerate the process of autophagy in your body significantly. You can accelerate your autophagy processes by skipping your breakfast and then eating generally within eight hours. This kind of fasting will Kickstart and stimulate your body's autophagy processes. Intermittent fasting also enables your body to do a cleanup on all the toxin build-ups in your body.

Moreover, when done effectively, intermittent fasting has been known to cause hormonal imbalance in women. This is because women are naturally susceptible to stressors, such as famine, through starvation or calorie restriction. The hormonal imbalance will then trigger off the process of autophagy. When you keep off any calories, you help your body to attain the fasting state. Your body will then communicate to your cells that it is starving, and the cells will automatically trigger the autophagy process.

Studies also show long fast promotes weight loss and autophagy. When you fast for 24 hours, your body will reverse any loss of stem function. This will enable your body to regenerate itself significantly.

If you are wondering how long you should fast in order to attain autophagy, then most studies agree that a 24-hour period is suitable, although other studies recommend a 16 hour period for your body to trigger autophagy. It has been found that the 16-hour fasting is not as effective as the 24-hour fasting when it comes to autophagy.

Exercising using high-intensity interval training

You can also stimulate your autophagy by engaging in high-intensity interval training. Such training exposes your body to stress, thus triggering autophagy. You should always remember that autophagy is a natural way through which your body responds to stress. High interval exercises put your body through so much stress that biochemical changes are automatically provoked. Engaging in top impact load exercises will not only make your muscles to be build up but also induce autophagy.

For optimal effect, aim at approximately 20 to 30 minutes of high impact exercises each day. Moreover, experts reckon that you should engage in weight lifting and resistance training exercises for at least 30 minutes each day for your body to effectively Kickstart the process of autophagy. Such exercise usually exposes your body to acute stress. Autophagy loves stress so that the process will be automatically triggered off.

Alternatively, you can engage in other practices involving brisk walking and slow pace walking. This exercise has also been shown to be good at triggering off your autophagy process. Remember to incorporate healthy eating and water intake to your workouts.

Get enough sleep

Studies show when you get enough sleep, the process of autophagy is highly boosted. Specifically, experts believe that you can activate your autophagy by adopting your body's natural clock or circadian rhythms or sleep-wake cycles. However, you need first to study the four sleep personalities to determine the therapeutic sleep cycle, which works best for you.

You should, therefore, avoid giving up your sleep for your favorite movies or work if you want the process of autophagy to be kick-started in your body.

Studies have revealed that your body works well when you respect its natural clocks or circadian rhythms. Your biological clock usually controls your sleep cycle and patterns. It also influences your autophagy process by controlling it.

When you respect your natural clock, your metabolism process is significantly boosted. While you are asleep, your body makes use of this time to produce and release beneficial hormones. When you deprive yourself of sleep; therefore, you subject it to undue stress, which may have adverse effects on your overall health.

Sleep is very critical in inducing autophagy in your body. Lack of sleep disrupts the process of autophagy or make the process to be prolonged.

Eat autophagy boosting foods

Certain foods help in accelerating the process of autophagy once you consume them. The following are some of the food that helps to induce your body's cleansing process:

Coffee- studies link coffee consumption to the reduction of incidence of metabolic diseases. Coffee is so effective in reducing the metabolic disease because it increases the autophagy process throughout your body. When you consume a single cup of coffee, it leads to a significant increase in autophagy in your liver, heart and muscle cells.

Ginger- consumption of ginger can dramatically increase your autophagy. Studies reveal the 6-shogaol components of ginger induces the process of autophagy. The autophagy induced by ginger is so powerful it can destroy a type of lung cancer cells.

Green tea-consuming green tea can help induce your autophagy. Green tea contains some active ingredients called EGCG, which plays a critical role in triggering the process of autophagy in your body. The process is beneficial in fighting inflammation, liver damage, and cancer.

Coconut oil- coconut oil contains several ketones. Ketones are the same components that you seek to produce when you engage in fasting. Consuming coconut oil, therefore, will induce autophagy without necessarily starving yourself.

Using autophagy to get rid of stubborn fats

You can manipulate autophagy to lose stubborn fats in your body. However, you need to understand what triggers the process first. You should also be willing to make the necessary lifestyle for autophagy to work well in helping you to lose the stubborn fats.

When you alter your diet, you help autophagy to fine-tune its processes to effectively get rid of excess fats and make your metabolic processes to be more efficient.

Autophagy can be used to trick your metabolism into working for many hours to burn more fat. The key advantage of this method is that it tends to work at cellular levels and thus produces better and faster results.

For autophagy to work best in increasing your weight loss, you need to incorporate intermittent fasting. This means that you eat a well-planned out diet during a specific window period, and for the rest of the day, you engage in severe fasting for your body to burn the excess fats.

However, before you engage in autophagy fasting, you should seek your doctor's advice on the best diet to follow to achieve better results.

What SLEEP Got To Do With It

Circadian rhythms and sleep are very important to maximize autophagy. Circadian rhythms refer to the physiological processes of the body that connect with the day and night cycles of your surroundings. The rhythms control the brain, epigenetics, and hormones. Misaligned rhythms are always associated with obesity, diabetes, metabolic syndrome, cancer, depression, and neurodegeneration. This is usually caused by exposure to evening light, which interferes with the circadian clock, and interferes with the quality of sleep.

Deprivation of sleep and poor sleep quality can cause negative health impacts, including Alzheimer's, diabetes, mood disorders, decreased performance, and increased dying risks. Getting quality sleep is the most important means of having a healthy life.

Autophagy and Sleep

When sleeping, the body undergoes important physiological processes like physical repair, memory consolidation, muscle growth, fat loss, learning new skills, and autophagy. This is the moment when the brain clears out toxic proteins and beta-amyloid, which are associated with autophagy.

Having quality sleep is very crucial in maximizing the benefits of autophagy. The sleep hormone, melatonin, is the one that modulates autophagy. On the other hand, autophagy is also important to get better sleep.

Up to 70% of the pulses of growth hormones happen during deep sleep. The hormones facilitate regeneration, fat burning, and physical repair. The growth hormones stimulate the liver to initiate autophagy while also supporting the production of glucose.

Can one still gain autophagy with poor sleep? To an extent, gaining autophagy without sleep or with poor sleep quality is possible. However, poor sleep might cause several health conditions. Also, misaligned circadian rhythms also cause stress on the body, thereby preventing one from staying healthy. Nevertheless, restricted feeding within 6 to 8 hours can actually improve one's quality of sleep due to the increased basal level of autophagy.

Chapter 3: How To Achieve Autophagy

Boosting autophagy in your body simply means trying to make your body operate at its optimum. You are maximizing your output and increasing your body's efficiency. Amazingly, not only is your body operating at its maximum, but it is operating on clean energy . You can call this the body's version of green energy. You are supplying your body with nutrients and energy in the cleanest (healthiest) way possible.

There are three major ways to boost autophagy in the body.

Keto diet

This is a simple and natural way of activating autophagy without forgoing some of your favorite meals. The idea is to reduce carbohydrate levels. When carbohydrate levels are low, the body has no choice but to use fat as a fuel source. This is the concept behind the extremely popular ketogenic diet.

Keto diets are diets high in fat and low in carbohydrates (e.g. teak, bacon and peanut butter shakes). Between 60 and 70 percent of your overall calories come from fat. Proteins are the next major contributors. They make up about 20 to 30% of the body's calories.

Protein provides 20 to 30 percent of calories, while only 5 percent comes from carbs. This shows that carbohydrates are the most insignificant part of our diet. While proteins can be converted into sugar (in the absence of carbohydrates), fats cannot.

So basically, in ketosis you lose excess body fat while retaining muscle. Ketogenesis equally aids the body in resolving cancerous tumors, lowers the risk of diabetes and protects the body from brain disorders such as epilepsy. Ketosis can be said to be an autophagy hack. Through keto-diets you can gain the benefits of autophagy, without stressing your body too much. In keto-diets there is a gradual shift from burning carbs (glucose) to ketones. Autophagy is keto-based, hence very little carb is involved in autophagy.

Fasting

-Water Fasting

Water fasting is a milder form of fasting. Fasting (in all forms) is one of the most effective ways of achieving autophagy. An individual undergoing a water fast can drink water. Although he or she will not consume anything else except water for twenty-four hours, water fasts might not be as effective as a full fast. A full fast does not involve water. Nothing is eaten within twenty-four hours. Water fasting benefits include weight loss, body cleansing, cellular regeneration and, most importantly, autophagy. It is increasing in popularity.

Also, the presence of oxygen in the water helps the body. It assists the body in eliminating harmful toxins. That is why water fasting is nicknamed the expert cleanser. Whenever water and fasting meet, detoxification must occur.

Water is calorie-free. That is why water enhances metabolism and ketogenesis. There are links between drinking water and weight loss. As the body shifts to ketosis during water fasting, it can use up excess fat. Water fasting also boosts the body's healing process. It reduces inflammation in the body and lowers blood sugar levels while enhancing the activities of the heart and brain. Additionally, drinking water supports collagen synthesis in the skin.

Tips (on water fasting)

Fasting requires a lot of effort. Before you begin a water fast, you need to prepare yourself mentally. You need to always picture the light at the end of the tunnel. Visualizing your goals will help motivate you.

Before commencing your water fast, you should have a doctor's consultation to decide the duration of your program.

Abstaining from food for a week and taking nothing but water can be very tough especially at the beginning. You might feel hungry or weak as your body will be in a state of ketosis after 3-4 days. The body adapts to this 'new' system and the fasting process becomes much easier.

Setting the duration of your fast

Fasting essentially means abstinence from all foods. In Islam or Christianity for example, fasting dates are based for days of the week, months or a year. It can be done for different durations.

Water fasting can last for as little as 3 days to a whole month based on the objective and capability7 of the person. For example, it is suggested that individuals suffering from chronic illnesses should avoid water fasts longer than 3 days.

The amount of water taken in a day is directly related to the individual's level of activity. Although the amount of water taken in is not critical (in respect to results), most people, irrespective of the amount of water they drink, experience tremendous changes (weight loss, detoxification, autophagy, etc.).

-Skipping meals/intermittent fasting

Skipping meals is another method you can use to achieve autophagy. Unlike ketosis, this method is stressful. At first you might not understand the benefits, but you are bound to become addicted once you start seeing the results. Recent studies have shown that periodic fasting and autophagy can make cancer treatments more productive. Normal body cells are not affected unlike in normal cancer therapy. Modern cancer therapies are very harsh. They make wholesale changes to your body size (weight) and can even affect your looks.

Recent research has shown that intermittent fasting improves brain function, brain structure and neuroplasticity. It helps the brain to reorganize and replenish itself. It equally helps to improve cognitive function and structures.

Intermittent fasting is simply taking skipping meals to another level. Intermittent fasting should be adopted to suit your capabilities and personal targets. Whichever way you choose to practice it, you are bound to reap some amazing benefits. Some of these benefits include increased resistance to diseases and infection, reduced body weight, increased lifespan, improved cardiovascular function, increased brain function and a whole lot more.

Children, pregnant women, people with ulcers, low sugar levels and persons with food associated ailments (diseases) are advised to practice intermittent fasting mildly. In some cases, they should avoid it totally, most especially pregnant women.

So then, the question is: *How can intermittent fasting improve autophagy?* Well let's compare this to a packed fridge. This fridge belongs to Mr. Food (hypothetic). He keeps packing his fridge with food. The fridge is now in layers (layers of food). Some of these foods reach their expiry dates. Mr. Food can't see or notice this. Naturally, decomposition begins, followed by a foul odor. Cool story, right?

This mirrors what happens in our bodies when we keep over feeding. The body is packed up with digestion products (glucose, fat, amino acids) that keep piling up. There's a popular adage: "too much of anything is never good". This is a universal truth. Our bodies, the atmosphere, water, soil, etc., all exist on a delicate balance. Nature finds a way to balance itself. No excesses, just perfection!

Intermittent fasting is one of the ways we can help our body to achieve this balance. Fasting forces the body to use up its stores. Some cells die during this process (autophagy). These cells are replaced by the body when you feed again. *Hence, the body is renewed and refreshed!*

-Longer fasts (no food or water)

Intermittent fasting is a vital tool for improving health, achieving weight loss, detoxification, cellular regeneration and autophagy. There is enough evidence to back this up. However, longer fasts have proven to be more effective. *Please, always fast according to your capabilities. You can achieve similar results with both water fasts, intermittent fasts and full fasts.*

Full fasting can take many forms. The most drastic is a "dry fast", which entails avoiding all edibles and fluids (food or water). Never start a full fast without consulting a medical practitioner. Full fasts can be very severe and shouldn't be done for more than 48 hours.

Long fasts and autophagy

The most outstanding benefit of full fasts is their ability to induce autophagy. If you abstain from food, your body will be forced to use up its stores. Old cells are recycled as well. They are used to build new cells (autophagy). After 24 hours, the body uses up most of the glycogen in the liver.

In respect to weight loss, the body loses around 1-2 pounds a day. This happens because it is shedding water weight and protein. However, the body's dependence on protein as a source of energy is short-lived. Using protein would mean breaking down muscles, some of which might be essential/delicate.

This makes fat a more reliable/suitable energy source. Hence, after a few days, the body switches to its fat stores for energy (ketosis). Fat is more energy-dense per pound than protein, so weight loss in this phase is slower. It reduces to just over 1 pound every 2 days.

A long fast is the easiest way of staying in ketosis for an extended duration. It forces the body to rely completely on its own fat stores instead of dietary fat. Being in ketosis makes weight loss easy. Ketosis helps suppress hunger (especially after the first few days, which are usually tough). Fasting also enables you to totally get your mind off food. It saves you the stress of thinking about what to eat next and bothering on the amount of food you are eating.

Full fast is an effective means to lose a lot of weight quickly. However, many people begin to gain it all back again because they just go back to their old eating pattern.

Like most "crash diets," fasting will help you lose weight, but won't help you maintain the status quo, unless you also make permanent changes in your diet after the fast is over.

As we noted earlier, long fasts promote autophagy, which can be compared to "spring cleaning" for your cells. Since the body is basically eating itself, it has a chance to eliminate any junk or waste products that may have built up, and repair the harm caused by oxidative stress. This is one of the substantial benefits of fasting even for people who have a healthy weight. Autophagy also has powerful anti-aging and muscle-building properties.

Recent research has shown that an extended fast (10 days on average) was beneficial to people suffering from hypertension, also noting that even though the patients didn't start the fasting program to lose weight, all of them had an average weight loss of around 15 pounds. Full fasts (up to 5 days) may also have some benefits for chemotherapy patients.

Another effect of full fasts is mental clarity. It is a way to break free from overeating patterns or other food disorders. Fasting is practiced by many religious groups because it enhances meditation and mindfulness. Briefly put, fasting declogs the mind and increases focus.

Exercise

Working out stresses the muscles (damages them in a good way). The muscles are torn and rebuilt. This makes them stronger and more resistant. Increasing your muscular strength improves your body's condition. People who exercise regularly are less prone to diseases and infections. Researchers have discovered that exercise improves the human immune system. Resistance training is usually the most effective type of exercise, not just for autophagy, but the body as a whole. When done at intervals, the body's conditioning improves. You tear up your muscles, rebuild stronger ones and stimulate autophagy.

Exercise is in essence a physical method of achieving autophagy. You use up your body stores directly when you exercise. Most people describe exercise as refreshing. Well, that is not just a feeling. It is actually happening. *Exercise catalyzes regeneration* (development of new cells). To regenerate means to replace lost or damaged tissue. So not only are new cells being produced, old ones are encouraged to die.

Exercising is very important in the treatment of any disease. How rigorous the exercise is, depends on your doctor's approval. Exercise improves your body's use of insulin and may lower blood sugar levels apart from helping to use up some of the excess glucose. Exercise equally helps to increase blood circulation, enhance kidney function, reduce risk of developing diabetes and in general helps to improve the body's condition.

Exercise can equally lower the chance of having a heart attack or stroke and can improve circulation. Furthermore, it has been proven that exercise benefits the brain greatly. It increases blood circulation to the brain and helps increase the brain's efficiency. Exercise is highly recommended, especially for those who are obese/overweight. Care should be taken not to over work the body in one go. Exercise should be gradual and progressive. A minimum of 150 minutes a week (total exercise time) is recommended.

A large number of diseases target and attack the muscles. They reduce their mass, finally rendering them useless. The body cannot function without strong muscles. Exercising daily helps your body keep its muscles alive and strong.

You do not have to follow a drastic, severe exercising program. All you have to do is try to exercise at least three hours a week. Walking in a park for an hour, running on a treadmill, going to the mall for three hours, in other words simply walking around often is a good start to keep your body in shape. When you go shopping, try to park far from the entrance so you have to walk more on your way there and back.

Exercising helps your blood circulate through your body and helps your body burn fat and bad calories. By exercising, the sugar in your blood is used to help your muscles function and therefore not be stagnant in vour organs and arteries. It is a simple process: more you eat, more you need to exercise and more you exercise, more you need to eat.

According to doctors and researchers, exercising is the best way to fight disease. However, it does so with a daily routine or at least a tri-weekly habit. Just walking around the block once a month is not enough, extra effort is needed.

Exercising helps you feel better about yourself as it releases endorphins in your body, the same endorphins you would get by eating your favorite food. Working out fights the high level of cholesterol and keeps cholesterol related diseases away.

If you plan on exercising daily and at a high level, talk about it with your doctor. He will help you find the best program for your needs and physical and medical abilities. You will have to take it slowly, step by step. Do not try to run a marathon on the first day or go on a five-mile run because you want to burn the calories. You will burn as many calories walking a mile at a good pace as you would by running the same distance.

Dietary tips

To achieve autophagy, you can try some of these dietary tips. At least once or twice a week, you should limit your protein intake to 15-25 grams a day. This gives the body nearly a day to recycle stored proteins, reduce inflammation and cleanse body cells. The best part is that the muscle mass remains the same. It does not shrink or reduce. During this abstinence period (food abstinence), the body is forced to consume its stored proteins and toxins. Skipping breakfast (say twice a week), helps to promote autophagy in the body. It gives the body time to clean itself (eliminate lingering toxins).

Research has shown that about 30% of women respond to intermittent fasting more severely. To curb these effects, a fat-based breakfast is recommended. Basically, you are required to keep carbohydrates and fat from your meals (for a whole day). However, the quantity taken should be regulated. Fats are energy

Kings. Half of kilogram of fat gives three or four times more energy than proteins or carbohydrates of the same quantity. So, taking in a very small quantity of fat is usually more than enough. This way, you are not starving your body, while promoting autophagy.

Your daily meals have a direct effect on your body. Some foods, when consumed in large quantities are unhealthy, while others have minimal or no negative effects on the body. Therefore, managing what you eat, knowing the calorie content, the ingredients and how they affect your body is very important. Generally, three major classes of food appear in most of our meals or diets. They include carbohydrates, fats and proteins. Vegetables, fruits and fiber appear much less in meals and diets. To influence your health positively, an understanding of these food classes and their effects on the body is very important.

Carbohydrates

These are one of the most popular food classes. They exist as starches, sugar and fiber in foods such as grains, fruits, vegetables, milk products and sweets. They increase blood sugar levels and affect the body more than any other food. Therefore, knowing what foods contain carbohydrates and regulating the amount per meal is helpful for blood glucose control. Carbohydrates in your meal should come from healthy sources like vegetables, fruits, whole grains and legumes. Also, carbohydrates coming from whole grain (high fibers) are recommended. Those originating from sources 'with added sugars, fats and salt should be avoided.

Carbohydrate control and regulation is the bedrock to achieving autophagy. Eating carbohydrates is not bad (unhealthy) in essence. The quantity simply has to be reduced, and carbohydrates from healthier sources should be integrated into meal plans. Eating carbohydrates from healthy sources can equally help you to lose excess body weight and generally make you healthier.

Proteins

Proteins are an important part of our diet. In an experiment where an individual consumed a given quantity of protein and another consumed the same quantity of carbohydrates, the individual who took the carbohydrates was most likely to be hungry first. This shows how important proteins are in helping create satiety. Proteins mildly contribute to the glucose (sugar levels) in the body and are usually increased in most recommended meal plans (health meal plans). However, to achieve autophagy, proteins are not needed in high quantities. Proteins are equally the building blocks of the body, and generally help the body to recover from stress and ailments.

Fats

These are the number one energy givers in the body. Fats are an important component in the creation of balanced diets, and more importantly, in achieving autophagy. When digested, fats undergo ketosis (an important energy cycle the body experiences in times of starvation). Therefore, when you take the right amount of fats, you can induce artificial starvation. Most especially healthy fats are from fish (e.g. trout and salmon), nuts, seeds, olive oil, canola oil, other vegetable oils, avocado, and soft margarine. Fats don't raise blood glucose but are high in calories. Their high calorie content and energy giving ability7 means that very small quantities can sustain the body. Health wise, it is advisable to use non-saturated fatty acids as against saturated fatty acids. Sources of saturated fatty acids include butter, red meat, cakes, pastries and deep-fried foods. Instead, plant-based protein and lower fat dair\' products should be used more often.

Generally, to create an autophagy inducing diet, fats should be included more in the diet, albeit in differing quantities.

Vegetables and fruit

Vegetables and fruits are beneficial to the body. They help in flushing and cleansing the body. They contain many vitamins and minerals to help supply vital nutrients and regulate vital body activities. They can equally be used as snacks, because most of them contain fibers. Hence, they can easily cause satiety. Fruits also contain natural sugars which are less harmful to the body.

Other methods to induce autophagy

-Drugs

Although the use of drugs to achieve autophagy is still relatively untested (in its infancy), certain drugs have the ability to induce autophagy. Although their actions are usually specific (inducing their effects in certain parts of the body), their actions are not generalized.

For example, latrepirdine, resveratrol and lithium are used to stimulate autophagy in patients with Huntington's disease. Since research is presently ongoing, their usage is still very limited.

In the treatment of Alzheimer's disease, certain drugs/substances such as nicotinamide, hydroxy chloroquine, resveratrol, nilotinib, lithium, latrepirdine, metformin, valproic acid and statins have been credited with inducing different levels of autophagy. Equally, in the treatment of Parkinson's disease nilotinib and statins have been credited with inducing autophagy. Lastly, lithium, tamoxifen, and valproic are said to be capable of inducing Amyotrophic lateral sclerosis (ALS).

Most of these drugs are relatively untested. However, advancements are being made as we speak. Their usage is currently limited to neurodegenerative and auto-immune diseases. In the future, it is hoped that autophagy would be more widely used.

-Regulating sleep

It is recommended that we get at least 7-9 hours of sleep a day. Despite these recommendations, modern research has shown that the amount of sleep an individual requires depends on his or her sleep personality. This factor is scientifically called the sleep chronotype. Studies have shown that about 4 sleep personalities exist. Each sleep personality requires a certain amount of sleep a day (different sleep combinations). Certain individuals (based on their sleep personality) can cope with less sleep, while others require more. Sleep plays an important role in body recovery (regeneration of cells). Therefore, knowing the exact amount of sleep you need per day is very important. However, it should be noted that sleep is qualitative and not quantitative. Sleeping for hours under duress and in uncomfortable conditions might not be beneficial for the body. Less hours of sleep in a comfortable and relaxed environment, position or place might be worth more.

-Drink coffee

Modern research has shown that caffeine can induce autophagy in the muscle tissue, liver and heart. Even when taken on a full stomach or with other foods, its ability to induce autophagy is not reduced.

-Turmeric

Turmeric has proven to be effective in inducing autophagy in the cell, specifically in the mitochondria. This is majorly due to curcumin, a nutrient found in turmeric.

-Virgin olive oil

Virgin olive oil contains an antioxidant called oleuropein. Oleuropein is said to have anti- cancerous properties, one of which stems from its ability to induce autophagy.

-Ginger

Ginger consumption can help induce autophagy. This is because ginger contains an active component called 6-shogaol. 6-shogaol has become renowned for its efficiency in the treatment of lung cancer.

-Green Tea

The ingredient responsible for the autophagic ability of green tea is called polyphenol. It is found in both green and white tea. It is organ-specific, with most of its actions focused on the liver, where it helps to prevent inflammation, cancer and liver damage.

-Coconut Oil

Coconut oil is rich in ketones. Ketones are natural components produced by the body in times of starvation. Hence, by taking coconut oil, you are inducing starvation (a fake one) in the body.

-Reishi Mushroom

Even before its autophagy inducing properties where discovered, Reishi mushrooms where used in traditional medicine for decades in Asia. Modern research has shown that Reishi mushrooms can induce autophagy, which in turn produces anticancer effects in those who suffer from breast cancer.

-Vitamin D

Also known as the sunshine vitamin, vitamin D is synthesized naturally in the body (specifically in the skin). Its precursors are activated by sunlight. Those staying in regions where sunlight is minimal or non-existent (e.g. artic regions) might have to take synthesized vitamin D.

Vitamin D is capable of inducing autophagy in the pancreatic islets. Predictably, this will increase insulin production in the pancreas and is therefore helps prevent cancer. very effective in the treatment of type 2 diabetes.

-Melatonin

Melatonin is the only hormone on this list. It plays an important role in the regulation of our circadian rhythm (circadian rhythm is very important in coordinating sleep). Recent studies have shown that melatonin supplementation can induce autophagy in the brain. It helps to protect the brain from cell injury. Cellular injury is one of the leading causes of neuropsychiatric conditions around the world.

-Ginseng (ginseng root)

Ginseng is one of the most important natural supplements in the world today. It is sold around the globe and is even capable of boosting the human immune system. Apart from its immune boosting ability, it also induces autophagy and

Chapter 4: How To Induce Autophagy?

"Fasting of the body is food for the soul"

Saint John Chrysostom

Autophagy Fasting

Also called the process of restricting the intake of calories for a period of time, fasting brings some remarkable health benefits. From weight loss, low risks of diabetes, a serious cardiovascular complication to a longer life, fasting can play a crucial role.

Over the years, researchers have been trying to determine the reasons why fasting is linked to longevity. Studies indicate that mice and monkeys that undergo fasting are likely to live longer than regularly fed peers.

Research finds that calorie restriction turns on a gene that tells cells to preserve their resources. Particularly, the cells go into a famine mode, making them resistant to cellular stress and diseases. From there, they enter the process of autophagy in which the body starts to clean out unwanted cellular materials.

A **study** about mice that fasted for a day indicated a number of autophagosomes – a sign that autophagy is working. But take note that a mouse's metabolism is faster compared to human metabolism. Although it is complicated to measure autophagy outside a laboratory, the process initiates in a person after at least 18 hours of fasting. The maximum benefits, however, occur after 48 or 72 hours. It sounds daunting, isn't it? The good news is that the intermittent fasting results in several benefits. To stimulate autophagy and clean damaged cells, a longer fasting can be a smart idea. But it's ideal to consult a qualified physician before anything else.

Autophagy stimulation can clear out old cellular materials, activate a good level of growth hormones, regenerate fresh cells, and shorten cell renewal. Autophagy can also destroy viruses and other lingering bacteria, which are common to people who suffer from an infection.

Aside from increasing longevity, autophagy has been linked to Alzheimer's, Parkinson's, and other degenerative diseases. As autophagy does not take place, the body collects a range of cellular material. This includes a protein that comes in a large quantity in patients with cancer and degenerative illnesses. Specialists believe that a prolonged process of autophagy might increase the possibility of clearing the brain from excess proteins. Therefore, preventing the development of such diseases is possible.

With the underlying health benefits of autophagy, a large number of drug companies have been trying to develop a pharmaceutical panacea to activate the process. There are also fitness and diet bloggers who claim that supplements can lead to autophagy. But it still requires extensive research to prove the claim.

Generally, fasting is a proven way to induce autophagy. When a person's nutrients become depleted, autophagy involves two pathways, such as mTOR and AMPK. Called as mammalian target of rapamycin, MTOR regulates the nutrients that affect anabolism, protein synthesis, and even cellular growth. It has also been linked to the stimulation of new tissue creation and insulin receptors.

AMPK, on the other hand, stimulates the body's backup fuel mechanisms and maintains energy homeostasis. Both mTOR and AMPK are attuned to the nutrients available in the body. These two pathways aid the body to decide whether it will go into autophagy or stimulate a growth response.

Autophagy also works with insulin and glucagon. Patients with hypoglycemia and diabetes experience a hard time regulating insulin. As glucagon goes up, the insulin goes down and vice versa. When a person undergoes intermittent fasting, the insulin drops while the glucagon increases.

However, it's easier said than done to induce autophagy. It is also important to have a low liver glycogen, which is achieved after 14 hours of fasting. But not everyone has the same needs. For some patients, they achieve low liver glycogen after 24 hours. The secret here is a serious commitment, discipline, and patience.

Despite the benefits, fasting is not suitable for everyone. Some patients experience mood swings, low-energy, insomnia, and other complications.

Autophagy Exercise

Aside from intermittent fasting, exercise can induce autophagy.

For multiple decades, the number of people with diabetes, cancer, or cardiovascular complications has been growing. While medical experts develop an FDA approved and new treatment, exercise is one of the best ways to alleviate such an alarming rate.

Scientifically speaking, the human body is built to move. Most people, however, don't perform on a regular basis due to a busy lifestyle, health issues, and other special conditions.

Proper and regular exercise has been shown to fight cancer cells as it boosts autophagy, just like intermittent fasting.

Before, experts conducted clinical trials to detoxify people from the Gulf War. Results indicated that a combination of exercise, niacin supplementation, and sauna eliminated toxins from the body. But wait, there's more! A simple or strenuous workout routine increases vasodilation and blood flow.

Recently, scientists have engineered mice to have green autophagosomes. They found that the mice demolished their cells after a 30-min run on a treadmill. The rate also increased, especially when they ran past the 30-minute mark.

Exercise specifically induces autophagy in the brain's peripheral tissues. While lab mice without exercise can't run on a treadmill, wild-type mice are different. They gained a glucose uptake through muscles. Autophagy also supports the growth of new brain cells after a simple exercise.

Exercise can help restore failing autophagy in a heart tissue with a damage. Autophagy targets dysfunctional mitochondria and other damaged areas that increase the risks of oxidative stress and inflammation.

Where is mitochondria located? More than the liver and heart, it is available in the brain and other vital organs. With regular exercise, the body can lessen the risk of developing dysfunctional mitochondria. Thanks to autophagy.

Autophagy also promotes aerobic performance. This is especially true when a patient takes a high-altitude training. Aside from stimulating autophagy, hypoxia is known to increase blood flow.

Intermittent fasting stimulates the AMPK pathway. Exercise is no exception. As soon as it activates the AMPK pathway, autophagy comes next. In the previous chapter, we understand that AMPK regulates the breakdown pathways and protein synthesis. But it goes beyond that. In fact, it comes into play in skeletal muscle homeostasis.

AMPK also serves as a regulator of skeletal muscle protein turnover. What is a protein turnover? Simply, it's the balance between protein breakdown and build-up within the day. When does a person become in a more anabolic state? It's when the protein synthesis surpasses the amount of protein breakdown.

Autophagy supports skeletal muscle plasticity in response to any endurance workout. Unlike a fed state, exercise performed in a fasted condition increases LC3B-II. To have a better autophagic response, a combination of intermittent fasting and exercise provides a stronger effect. Also, someone taps straight into his body fat for enough source of energy.

Low-intensity cardio and aerobic exercise also burn ketones and fat for fuel, enabling the body to produce energy from fat. That means an individual can continue hitting the gym within a long period of time.

However, strenuous exercise can activate excessive autophagy, resulting in catabolism and muscle atrophy. Too much energy deprivation also affects anabolic growth and prevents a fast recovery.

The key here is to stimulate specific regions. Start from the brain, liver, heart, kidneys, or adipose tissue to recycle damaged or dysfunctional cells. Instead of too much autophagy in the muscles, increase the level of mTOR.

With intermittent fasting and resistance training, a patient can stimulate MTOR and autophagy as well.

High-intensity interval training (HIIT) is another ideal way to activate autophagy. Bear in mind that the latter is a response to stress. With a high-intensity exercise, it puts you in a good-stress sweet state. A person can get sufficient impact load, which in turn makes the muscles stronger without any health dangers. A HIIT that lasts for at least 20 minutes can promote longevity and boost confidence.

Autophagy Diet

In the previous chapter, we understand that autophagy means "self-eating." So, it makes sense that ketogenic and intermittent fasting diets have been a popular way to trigger autophagy. Which is better? Fasting is a more effective way, according to experts. Ketosis, on the contrary, is like a shortcut that results in some metabolic changes.

What's a ketosis? It's simply a diet that's low in carbs and high in fat. With proper ketosis, everyone can experience the same benefits of fasting. It particularly gives the body an opportunity to focus on its own repair and optimal health. But providing the body with an overwhelming load can change everything. The right amount of load can come into play, according to specialists.

Unlike the other popular diets, keto allows everyone to get at least 75% of calories from fat and 5% of calories from carbohydrates. Over time, this causes the body to change metabolic pathways. Rather than glucose from carbs, it starts to use fat for energy. From there, it begins to produce ketone bodies, which provide strong protective effects. Recent studies show that ketosis triggers starvation-induced autophagy. That's not all! It has some neuroprotective functions.

A low level of glucose occurs in intermittent fasting and keto diet. It has also been linked to a high glucagon and low insulin. The latter triggers autophagy.

The keto diet also activates the pathways that intermittent fasting stimulates. AMPK pathway is a good example.

In rats, the diet triggered autophagy and protected its brain from any seizure-induced injury and other serious complications.

Diets are divided into several versions. Standards Ketogenic Diet (SKD), Targeted Ketogenic Diet (TKD), Cyclical Ketogenic Diet (CKD), and the high-protein ketogenic diet is the most common versions. SKD is low in carb and rich in fat. The protein is moderate. CKD involves a period of higher-carb refeeds. TKD allows everyone to add carbs during a workout routine. A high-protein ketogenic diet, on the other hand, is a standard one. As the name indicates, it is rich with more protein.

In a keto diet, there are specific foods to eat, including meat, fatty fish, eggs, cheese, healthy oils, avocados, low-carb veggies, butter, nuts, and more. For condiments, everyone can use pepper, salt, herbs, and spices.

There are some foods to avoid, such as grains, beans, root vegetables, and alcohol. It would be extremely beneficial to slowly incorporate a ketogenic type diet in your life to gain maximal benefits of autophagy. Dietary changes to a keto or plant base iet would allow you to experience the true value of autophagy.

Chapter 5: How Autophagy Works

Autophagy exists because it works. Autophagy is a way that our body can repair damaged tissues or components without having to resort to apoptosis. Apoptosis should be thought of as a last resort. Programmed cell death is what our body must turn to when its components are absolutely beyond salvation. But sometimes cells and tissues are capable of being repaired and recycled. Indeed, sometimes the problem is an individual cell or an individual protein. If the body can merely get rid of this bad component then it cannot only restore its function, but it can improve it by removing a weak link in the chain. When we remember that these broken down components are then used to build new ones, the underlying benefits of this process to a complex organism like a human being becomes obvious.

In this chapter, we will examine how autophagy works by exploring the three major types of autophagy, namely macroautophagy, microautophagy, or chaperone-mediated autophagy (or CMA). These types of autophagy frequently work together to achieve the desired metabolic or exercise effect, but occasionally they have individual roles, as is the case of the role of microautophagy in helping the cardiovascular system deal with the drug rapamycin. Understanding the different types is the beginning of understanding in more detail the complexity of autophagy and how this complexity can really be distilled into three simple tools: fasting, dieting, and exercise.

The three main types of autophagy discussed here generally involve the operation of well-known cellular organelles, such as the lysosomes, endoplasmic reticulum, ribosomes, and mitochondria, although lesser-known structures such as the autophagosome and phagophore will also be discussed. As with other chapters in this book, some aspects of detailed terminology are explained in the glossary for reference purposes. The reason for exploring this subject is not to inundate the reader with details, but to help them make connections that may be of use to them later when it comes to being better understanding.

The Basics

Autophagy is a housekeeping tool that involves several organelles working together to accomplish the goal of keeping the cellular house in order. This may mean removing components that are damaging to the cell-like free radicals, processing degradation products so they can be reused for energy or repurposed, and even deciding that the cell itself should be degraded because it no longer meets the needs of the organism (in this case, the human body). The basic unit of autophagy function has been traditionally regarded as the lysosome, but further studies in recent decades have revealed that this organelle takes a back seat to a structure called the autophagosome.

This is not to say that the lysosome is not important. This organelle is extremely important, both in terms of the autophagy process and in related pathways like apoptosis. The lysosome is a double membrane structure that contains enzymes and other protein complexes that are capable of degradation and signaling. This allows the lysosome to work alone for breakdown, although it typically works in concert with other organelles. The name of the lysosome literally means "breaking (or breakdown) body."

The lysosome receives components for a breakdown from a double membrane vesicle known as the autophagosome. The presence of a double membrane is important as it allows components from outside the cell to be introduced into the interior of the cell, and it also allows the autophagosome to fuse with the lysosome, which contains enzymes and other necessary components. The movement of the autophagosome to the lysosome for breakdown and recycling occurs via the movement of microtubules which pull the organelles this way or that. This is the basic foundation for most autophagy pathways.

Macroautophagy

Macroautophagy is a process that utilizes several steps to trap components in the cytoplasm and recycle them. The first step is the formation of a structure called the isolation membrane. The formation of this structure is triggered by specific factors, some of which will be discussed further shortly. This structure is formed within the cell's cytoplasm; that is, the "sea" of fluid within the cell, as opposed to extracellular fluid outside the cell membrane. Cells are very good at using membranes to separate extracellular components from intracellular ones. This is a means of regulating what is able to enter the cell and protecting the cell.

The second step after the formation of the isolation membrane is the formation of a structure known as the phagophore: a larger structure compared to the initial isolation membrane. The phagophore undergoes a process of expansion which leads to the engulfing of components in the cytoplasm and the formation of a third structure, the autophagosome. The autophagosome may be thought of as the basic essential structure of autophagy. This structure moves towards an important organelle called the lysosome, which results in the fusing of the autophagosome with the lysosome. The result is that the contents of the autophagosome are dumped into the lumen of the lysosome for degradation and recycling.

As it would be against the interests of our bodies to be degrading components willy nilly, macroautophagy is controlled in a highly nuanced manner by a series of triggers. Many of these triggers are in turn signaled and regulated by a number of proteins encoded in genes. Autophagy-related genes, or Atg, refer to proteins involved in the steps that lead to the formation of the autophagosome (via elongation).

Triggers of macroautophagy (in general terms) include:

- Fasting or starvation
- Lack of oxygen in the lungs
- Presence of reactive oxygen species
- Presence of infectious agents
- Therapeutic agents or drugs (like chemotherapy)

Microautophagy

In macroautophagy, the lysosome passively receives the vesicle (the autophagosome) containing the components intended for degradation and recycling. The autophagosome fuses with the lysosome in this case. In microautophagy, the lysosome is the main actor, directly engulfing the components in the cytosol that are intended for degradation. This process involves the double membrane of the lysosome folding in around the components that are being brought into the organelle, a process known as invagination. Like macroautophagy, this process is stimulated by specific triggers, of which factors in the environment are known to be significant.

Chaperone-mediated Autophagy (CMA)

Chaperone-mediated autophagy, or CMA, is an interesting pathway that is an active area of research. This type of autophagy also relies on the lysosome. In this pathway, particles designated for destruction are tagged with a molecule known as a chaperone. The chaperone is there to tag along, alerting the cell's organelles (particularly the lysosome), that this article is intended for destruction. The particle with the chaperone is recognized by receptors on the lysosomal membrane, which then invaginates the particle.

Other Types of Autophagy

There are several other types of autophagy that have been studied. Some of these fall under the three categories of macroautophagy, microautophagy, and chaperone-mediated autophagy, while others can be regarded as standalone pathways. For example, aggrephagy is regarded as a type of macroautophagy. Some lesser-known types of autophagy include.

Zymography: the detection and degradation of granules in the pancreas

Xenography: the degradation of toxic and infectious particles

Ribophagy: the breakdown of ribosomes

Pexography: the breakdown of peroxisomes (a type of organelle)

Mitophagy: the breakdown of mitochondria by lysosomes

Lipophagy: degradation of lipid droplets by autophagy

Chlorography: the protection from sunburn in some organisms

Aggrephagy: the degradation of cellular protein aggregates in macroautophagy

Autophagy Use in Therapeutic Agents

Autophagy has garnered attention in recent years for a number of reasons, not least of which is the potential use of autophagy as a target of therapeutic agents. That autophagy can be targeted for use by therapies for a wide number of purposes should come as a surprise to no one. Autophagy has already proven itself to be a tool that can be useful in cancer, weight loss, infection, and inflammation. In particular, autophagy has received attention for its potential uses in cancer.

Cancer therapies are often highly damaging to the person undergoing them.

Chemotherapy and radiation can damage normal cells right alongside the abnormal ones, forcing scientists to find ways to streamline these sorts of therapies in order to spare normal tissue as much as possible. But therapies based on autophagy work by different means, and they have the potential of doing very little harm to non-cancerous cell. This is a function of autophagy's role as an entirely normal cellular process in human beings, which places this pathway in juxtaposition to chemotherapy and radiation which are essentially toxic therapies designed to be used against cancerous cells.

There are two main roles that therapeutic agents that operate based on autophagy can play in cancer. The first role is the use of therapeutic agents that attempt to stimulate autophagy and remove cancerous or otherwise dysfunction cells. In this scenario, a drug would stimulate autophagy in a particular cell type (like hepatic cells, for example), which would lead to the body naturally clearing cancerous cells and their components in the liver. The second role may be a little counterintuitive to some. This second role would involve therapeutic agents to block autophagy and trigger apoptosis in the cell.

Blocking autophagy may seem like something that you would not want to do, but in the case of cancer cells, there is a reason to take this route. Autophagy is also used to preserve cells that may be damaged or exposed to damaging particles, like infectious particles or free radicals. Autophagy does not only remove malfunctioning cells, but it saves those cells that can and should be salvaged. By inhibiting autophagy in cancer cells, the body will be able to trigger apoptosis in these cells and clear them, which would theoretically result in the clearing of a cancerous tumor. Indeed, cancer cells have evolved numerous ways of preserving themselves using genes and one of these ways is to prevent apoptosis from being triggered in cancerous cells.

Recall the apoptosis is programmed cell death, and it can be triggered by a number of factors and thresholds in the cell. Essentially, these triggers are designed to lead to cell death when it is clear that the cell has passed a threshold where it can (or should) be salvaged. The body is able to recognize that rapidly replicating or otherwise dysfunctional cells like cancerous tumors are "bad" and should be removed by the body using apoptosis. The cancer cells block apoptosis, causing these cells to be preserved when they should not be. By blocking autophagy in these cells, therapeutic agents can push the balance in favor of apoptosis.

Naturally, understanding autophagy deeply requires an in-depth understanding of how it can be stimulated or encouraged. Now that you understand the benefits of autophagy and the major pathways through which it operates you can begin to explore the major ways to stimulate this important process. In the next chapter, you will learn more about the three major mechanisms by which you can encourage autophagy in your body and reap all of the benefits.

Chapter 6: Autophagy Through The Ketogenic Diet

Autophagy really kicks into high-gear when you're fasting, but it's difficult for most people to fast, even intermittently. What can be done instead? The ketogenic diet, a very popular diet these days, mimics many of the biological effects and benefits of fasting. In this chapter, we'll talk about what the keto diet is, how autophagy fits into the picture, and how to use the keto diet to trigger autophagy.

The history and science of the keto diet

The ketogenic diet wouldn't exist if it wasn't for epilepsy. Thousands of years ago, doctors figured out that seizures could be prevented by fasting. They didn't know why, but for some reason, it worked. Now, we know that fasting kickstarts autophagy, but it also kickstarts the production of liver compounds known as "ketones." Ketones are what most likely prevents seizures. For years, people fasted to prevent seizures, but doctors wanted to try something different. After some experiments with low-calorie diets, a doctor at the Mayo Clinic created the ketogenic diet, naming it after the ketones. This low-carb, high-fat diet triggered ketone production just like fasting. How?

Normally, when you eat a diet high in carbs, these get turned into glucose. That's the body's main source of fuel, and without any carbs, the body would die. However, when you significantly cut down on carbs and eat lots of fat in its place, the body is fooled into thinking it doesn't have any enough nutrients. It starts producing ketones for energy through the process of ketosis. Unlike glucose, excess ketones are not stored as body fat, which makes the keto diet a popular weight-loss diet. To trigger ketosis, a specific calorie division is needed. Your diet should consist of 5-10% carbs, 15-30% protein, and 60-70% fat. With the keto diet, you can mimic the effects of fasting, but without the actual starvation aspect.

Ketosis and autophagy

It's important to note that being in ketosos and being in autophagy are not mutally-exclusive. You can be in ketosis and not in autophagy, and vice versa. If you are really committed to autophagy through a keto diet, you need to be strict about your percentages. Stick to the highest fat and lowest carb percentage. Too much protein can also stop autophagy. You might also want to think about intermittent fasting in addition to a keto diet to consistently stay in autophagy. It's very easy to eat just a bit too much carbs or protein, and deactivate autophagy. Occasional fasting can keep that from happening. Over on writer and performance coach Siim Land's site, he also recommends using time-restricted eating (eating only at certain times of the day) and exercise in your keto diet for autophagy.

How can you tell if your keto diet is allowing you to achieve autophagy? You can't measure autophagy, but you can measure ketones, and they give you an idea of where you are with autophagy. There are three tools that can measure ketones: urine strips, a blood meter, or breath test. Urine strips measure specifically for acetoacetate, but they are only useful at the beginning of ketosis, because soon, the body starts using ketones and they aren't eliminated through pee. Breath tests measure for acetone. On its own, acetone isn't too important for ketosis, but levels of it tend to match beta-hydroxybutyrate (BHB), a more significant ketone. Blood meters, while the most expensive test, measure for BHB and are generally thought to be the most accurate tool.

To figure out if autophagy is working on a higher level, you'll be looking at the glucose ketone index. This can be measured with a ketone meter (like a breath test or blood meter) and glucose meter. Here's what to do:

Measure your readings for your glucose meter and ketone meter, writing down the numbers.

Divide your glucose number by 18 in order to translate the glucose measurement

of mg/dL into mmol/L, which is what ketones are measured in. If you aren't in the

United States, your glucose will already be measured in mmol/L, so skip this part.

Now, divide the number you got by your ketone number. You've got your GKI.

Generally, anything below 3 means you have a high ketone level and low glucose. 3-6 is moderate ketosis, and 6-9 means low ketosis. You want your GKI to be low for autophagy. While GKI isn't the only measurement for autophagy or ketosis, it is helpful and can help guide your other nutritional choices.

Benefits of the ketogenic diet

The keto diet, even when autophagy isn't triggered, has a host of possible benefits, including:

Easier weight loss

On the keto diet, you aren't putting away excess glucose as body fat, because you only eat what you absolutely need, and ketones don't accumulate in the body as fat. Many people find that losing weight becomes much easier, especially when combined with exercise. Eliminating "empty carbs" like white bread, junk food, and sweets also helps with weight maintenance.

More energy

With a diet high in carbs, most people experience bursts of energy followed by a crash. On the keto diet, energy is dispersed more evenly through the day thanks to steadier blood sugar levels. You aren't going on a rollercoaster of highs and lows anymore. Many high-fat foods like coconut oil, fish, and nuts also help with mental energy and clarity. It's easier to concentrate, even after a long day at work.

Better skin and hair health

Fat is known for its hydrating properties, so many keto dieters with skin and hair problems experience improvements. Hair is sleeker, shinier, and less dry, while skin is moisterized. The elimination of inflammatory foods like cow's milk can also help with acne and other skin issues.

Ketogenic diet risks

As a restrictive diet (you can find the list of food in the next section below), the keto diet comes with risks. There are three main issues:

Transitioning in ketosis can be miserable

When you cut out carbs so significantly, the body freaks out for a while. It needs a transition period to start burning fat and producing ketones. During this time, a lot of people experience flu-like symptoms, like headaches and fatigue. If you had a very carb-heavy diet before, the symptoms can be really uncomfortable. Expect the transition to last between 1-2 weeks, and if your symptoms keep you from your normal routines, add back in some nutritionally-sound carbs, like nectarines or sweet potatoes. This will slow down the ketosis process, but you'll feel better, and you'll be more likely to stick to the diet.

Restricted diets can lead to micronutrient deficiency

While you'll obviously get more nutrients on a keto diet than if you fasted, fasting does have an end date, while the keto diet doesn't. If you aren't careful, a long-term keto diet can lead to micronutrient deficiencies. This is a risk with any diet that cuts out entire food groups like whole grains. Many keto dieters are low in nutrients like fiber, sodium, and magnesium. Be sure to watch your nutritional intake and check in with a doctor if you experience health issues.

The keto diet can manifest into disordered eating

Besides nutritional defiencies, restrictive diets should all come with a warning tag about disordered eating. This is a psychological issue that people with histories of eating disorders and OCD should be aware of. When there are a lot of rules and regulations around eating, it can be easy to start getting obsessive and preoccupied with food. Instead of finding health and welness, you're just stressed all the time. Physical consequences of disordered include weight fluctuations, fatigue, and fainting, while emotional signs like fixtations on the "goodness" of a food and your body; avoiding social situations because of food; and food rituals are common. In the quest for ketosis and autophagy, you want to be careful to not let food rule your life.

Succeeding on the keto diet

If you decide that you do want to pursue autophagy through ketosis, there are certain foods you need to focus on, and certain ones to avoid. Here are two lists:

Food you can eat
Meat + seafood

All meats and seafood should be grass-fed, organic, wild-caught, etc, to get the most benefits from them.

Beef

Poultry

Eggs

Fish/shellfish

Organ meats/veal/goat/lamb/etc

Pork

Full-fat dairy

Most dairy is allowed on the keto diet, with the notable exception of cow's milk. It has too many carbs.

Cheese (brie, cheddar, mozzarella, parmesan, ricotta, etc)

Cottage cheese

Cream cheese

Dairy-free milk/nut milks

Heavy cream

Plain unsweetened Greek yogurt
Vegetables + fruit

All produce should ideally be organic, whenever you can get it. Most fruit has too many carbs for ketosis, so you're pretty limited.

Alfalfa sprouts

Avocados

Bell peppers

Berries

Bok choy

Broccoli

Button mushrooms

Cabbage

Cauliflower

Celery

Citrus fruits

Cucumber

Eggplant

Garlic

Kale

Lettuce

Onions

Parsley

Radishes

Sea vegetables

Spinach

Swiss chard

Tomatoes

Watercress

Zucchini

Nuts + seeds

Pretty much all nuts, seeds, and their butters are allowed on the keto diet, though in moderation, because it's very easy to eat too many and get kicked out of ketosis.

Almonds

Brazil nuts

Chia seeds

Flax seeds

Macadamia nuts

Nut butters

Pecans

Pumpkin seeds

Seed butters

Sunflower seeds

Walnuts

Fats + oils

Almond oil

Avocado oil

Cocoa butter

Coconut oil/coconut cream

Duck fat

Exra-virgin, cold-pressed olive oil

Ghee

<small>BEVERAGES</small>

Drink-wise, water will always be the best, but you are allowed some other unsweetened beverages and herbal teas.

Black coffee

Herbal tea

Unsweetened sparkling water + seltzers

Unsweetened coconut water

Water
Baking and cooking supplies:

You can bake on the keto diet, but you use certain low-carb supplies and no refined sugars. For cooking supplies like condiments, you just need to be sure it doesn't have refined sweeteners or gluten.

Almond flour

Baking powder/baking soda

Coconut aminos

Coconut flour

Erythritol/stevia blends

Fish sauce

Monk fruit extract or powder

Psyllium husk thickener

Sugar-free ketchup

Sugar-free yellow mustard

Vinegar (white, wine, and apple cider)

Foods you shouldn't eat

Food high in carbs, processed ingredients, and artifical ingredients kick you out ketosis and halt the autophagy process, so they need to be avoided. While you can get away with eating healthy, nutrient-dense foods like fruit (if you arrange the rest of your eating to accomodate the carbs), most processed foods and grain will always be too much.

All grain

Barley

Buckwheat

Corn

Oatmeal

Quinoa

Rice

Wheat

Wheat gluten

Processed meats

Deli meat

Grain-fed meats

Hot dogs

Sausages

Certain vegetables + fruit

Apples

Artichokes

Bananas

Carrots

Clementine

Corn

Dried fruit

Fruit jam

Fruit syrups

Grapes

Kiwi

Mangos

Pears

Pineapple

Potatoes

Squash

Sweet potatoes

Watermelon

Yams

Beans+ legumes

Black

Chickpeas

Fava

Kidney

Lentils

Peas

White

Low-fat + fat-free dairy

Butter substitutes

Low-fat cream cheese

Low-fat sour cream

Low-fat yogurt

Skim milk

Refined + artificial sweeteners

Agave

Aspartame

Cane sugar

Corn syrup

Equal

Maple syrup

Raw sugar

Saccharin

Splenda

Sucralose

White sugar

Certain oils

Canola

Corn

Grapeseed

Peanut

Sesame

Soybean

Sunflower

Chapter 7: Lifestyle And Food Choices That Help Activate Autophagy

Fasting is not the only diet or lifestyle solution that can help activate autophagy. There are other lifestyle choices that can help to activate this cell-cleansing process and applying all of them together will only increase the benefits you experience.

Exercise is another key component of autophagy activation. Exercise activates your body's energy burning systems and elevates your hormones. Even without fasting, a low-carb diet and an intense workout regime can induce ketosis and autophagy in the body. The ideal way to activate autophagy is to exercise while you fast. This may seem like an unhealthy way to "push" yourself, but exercising while your fast increases the rate at which your body burns through its sugar reserves and enters the fat-burning stages where autophagy is activated.

During ketosis, the body is able to directly access fatty acids to burn for energy. This is a very healthy and natural way to sustain your body through its workout regimen. It is triggered a stress-response in your body that activates autophagy in order to ensure cell survival throughout the period of "stress." In fact, because fasting and ketosis elevate your hormone levels, it's actually better for you to exercise while you're fasting if you want to build muscle (Fung, 2016).

To fully enjoy the benefits of autophagy, you must also follow a nutritious diet on days when you aren't fasting. First, a diet high in carbs or sugar will extend the time it takes for your body to burn through your sugar reserves, which delays the process of ketosis and inhibits autophagy. Second, a diet high in carbs or sugar will undo any of the growth and healing you experience during autophagy. Ingesting unhealthy foods that cause damage to the body and will cause your body to work that much harder to heal during the autophagy processes, and so will essentially undermine all of your hard work. Better still, even if you don't or can't fast, there are certain foods you can eat that will actually trigger the autophagy processes, even when your body isn't in ketosis (Whittel, 2018).

You also don't have to fast to enter ketosis. Changing your diet to exclusively eat foods that are high-fat low-carb, and cutting processed sugar out of your diet altogether can also cause your body to enter ketosis, especially after you have been on this kind of diet for a long while. Whether you choose to fast or not, Chapter Six includes a list of nutritious high-fat, low-carb foods, some of which have autophagy-triggering properties, and a list of high-carb foods that can block ketosis and autophagy.

Another important lifestyle component of autophagy activation is stress-management. Though autophagy is considered a "stress-response," it's triggered by physical or environmental stress, such as nutrient deprivation or increased physical activity. Psychological stress, otherwise known as anxiety, can actually prevent autophagy activation because it blocks ketosis. Extreme anxiety causes the body to release a chemical called cortisol.

This chemical causes your liver and muscles to release sugar into the blood in order to help the body deal with whatever the situation is that's causing you stress. If you are being chased by a murderer or are in the path of an oncoming truck, this sudden release of sugar reserves can make the difference between life and death. If you are late paying your rent, on the other hand, when your body burns through its sugar reserves, instead of naturally switching over to burning fat, it starts converting your muscle protein into sugar (Berg, 2017).

Elevated anxiety levels are a signal to the body that you are in some kind of emergency, and so it will continue to flood your blood with sugar until those anxiety levels have sufficiently decreased. Therefore, extreme levels of psychological stress will not only block ketosis and autophagy, but fasting in a state of anxiety can be extremely harmful to the body. Stress- management strategies like a regular sleep pattern and meditation are therefore essential to reaping the benefits of autophagy.

Chapter 8: The Importance Of Detox

Our bodies can detox themselves through natural processes in the livers, kidneys, skin and bowels and through autophagy. However, we can also take special steps to detox ourselves through our diets and other lifestyle changes. This chapter is dedicated to the reasons why you might want to consider taking further steps to detox yourself.

Detox diets have earned a reputation of being based upon frivolous pseudoscience but detoxing is an incredibly important process in our body. Our health is assaulted from all angles by toxins and pollutants; everything from caffeine and alcohol to air pollutants from industry waste, car exhaust, and cigarette smoke. Most of the things we eat, even foods we consider healthy, have small amounts of toxic substances within them. Yet we can also allow toxins to enter our bloodstream through the skin and through the air that enters our lungs. Regardless of their source, our body regularly needs to deal with all the nasty compounds and chemicals that end up in the body, otherwise, we can face corresponding nasty health consequences.

In the body, the liver and the kidneys are the organs responsible for dealing with toxins in the body. The kidneys filter toxins from the blood, whilst the liver breaks down toxins into substances that can be used by the body or passed without trouble. If the kidneys and liver are burdened with too many toxins or if they are not kept in good shape through a healthy lifestyle, they can be unable to deal with all the toxins in the body. This can cause a huge array of problems; anything from fatigue and general feelings of being unwell, to bloating and digestive problems and even liver disease.

Most detox diets are aimed at eating lots of foods that help keep the liver and kidney in tip-top shape, but there are also many other methods to keep these crucial organs healthy. Drinking lots of water – at least 6 to 8 glasses per day – allows any waste products of the liver and kidneys to easily pass through the body. Likewise, you should avoid smoking and second-hand cigarette smoke, which contains over 4,000 different chemicals, including 43 cancer-causing carcinogens.

Eating too much sugar also makes your liver unhappy. By now everyone knows how consuming too much sugar can contribute to diabetes and the various health issues associated with weight gain, but the effects of sugar on the liver remain an enigma to most. The liver has a very limited ability to metabolize sugar, with some dieticians suggesting that anything more than 6 teaspoons of added sugar is excessive. Any sugar that the liver cannot break down is stored as fat, and a build-up of fat in the liver can lead to a condition called fatty liver disease.

Fatty liver disease, in turn, can lead to more serious conditions as bodily pain, fatigue, weakness and cirrhosis of the liver. Most people who are overweight or obese are at increased risk of fatty liver disease and they may be suffering from the condition in its early stages when there are few explicit symptoms.

Caffeine is another common toxin that the body has to deal with regularly. Caffeine is commonly associated with coffee, but it is also present in most fizzy drinks chocolate and energy drinks. The liver interprets caffeine as a foreign chemical and it is broken down through a special pathway in the liver that deals with manmade and unfamiliar substances, which includes most medication. For this reason, heavy caffeine consumption should especially be avoided when also taking certain drugs, especially pain relief chemicals such as acetaminophen.

Moderate caffeine consumption isn't dangerous or even unhealthy, with some studies suggesting it has numerous benefits on the body. Nonetheless, for the purposes of cleansing the body of toxins and giving the liver a period of relief, it's best to avoid this energy-booster or at least cut down on your silent addiction.

Good liver health can also be maintained by eating a diet rich in anti-oxidants which aid processing the waste products of toxins. Common antioxidants include vitamin C, vitamin E, beta-carotene, and zinc. Foods which are rich in anti-oxidants include dark chocolate, legumes, blueberries, red grapes, nuts, dark green veg, orange vegetable and green tea.

You can also help detox through eating organic food whenever possible. Non-organic foods are free from pesticide residue that may be left on non-organic foods. Many pesticides can build up in the human body and may be dangerous in noticeable concentrations. Eating organic, however, isn't always possible, practical or affordable, so sometimes it may be necessary to compromise. In general, if you eat the outer surface of grown food, it's more important that it is organic. Fruit such as strawberries, apples, grapes, cherries and leafy greens should preferably be organic, whereas with fruit or veg with peel it is less important (such as bananas and onions). The easiest way to detox your body is always to avoid toxins in the first place!

There is also a detox method you might not expect; getting more sleep. The western world has an embarrassing relationship with sleep. Sleep is vital for our well-being in dozens of different ways – it's where we rest our minds and rejuvenate our body. Yet all too many people resent their need to sleep and try to cheat themselves out of an hour or two every night. This can take a serious toll on well-being.

In terms of detoxing and cleansing the body, most of the detox process occur during sleep. In the resting state of sleep, your body is free to use resources and act in ways it simply can't when you are awake. For example, one of the main purposes of sleep is to filter toxins out of the brain; toxins which naturally as a side effect of being awake. The filtering system is called the lymphatic system and it is thought to be 10 times more activate during sleep, than during wakefulness. During sleep, numerous other metabolic processes take part, such as those which occur in the liver and are inhibited whilst active.

Whilst it might be rather obvious it is also worth mentioning that you can prevent toxins from getting into your system by avoiding places and environments where there are toxins present. Exhaust fumes, second-hand smoke and low air quality from industrial pollution are the main culprits, but depending on your location and career you may come into contact with many other types of toxins such as chemical residue from working in a factory, for example.

You can also aid the detox process by taking certain supplements, most notably milk thistle. Milk thistle is a small plant that grows in Mediterranean regions. It can be used as a herb and it also goes by the names Mary Thistle or Holy Thistle. Milk thistle is a popular natural choice for helping treat liver conditions such as cirrhosis or jaundice and it is also a staple of the detox community.

The active ingredient in milk thistle is called silymarin and it has powerful anti-inflammatory properties as well as being an anti-oxidant. Research on silymarin is still progressing and it's not entirely clear how it affects the body. Some studies have suggested that silymarin can aid liver function in individuals who have been exposed to industrial toxins, such as xylene and there is evidence to help it also improves type 2 diabetes and lowers cholesterol.

Finally, you can also try a temporary cleansing diet. Ultimately, our body needs the right materials to detox and as you might now understand, our regular diets don't give us enough resources to work with. You can rectify this by trying a cleansing diet intended to give your body a huge boost of all the vitamins, minerals, and good stuff it needs to cleanse itself.

Of course, ideally, a healthy, balanced diet will help the body cleanse itself over time and be exposed to fewer toxins. However, whether it's due to personal fault or factors beyond our control, we can't always consume a perfectly healthy diet. It might just be too pricey, we might not have the time or we might constantly be around other people who influence or control our eating habits.

Therefore, as a temporary solution or as a compromise you can periodically embrace a cleansing detox diet. These types of diets aren't intended to be a permanent change to your eating patterns and you shouldn't follow them for any period longer than 1-week. However, with that being said, they can give your body a reprieve to repair and rejuvenate itself, a benefit which can last for a few weeks or months before being required once more.

There are many different types of cleansing and detox diets, most of which involve consuming a large amount of fruit, vegetables, and calorie-free drinks. Try one out for a week and see how you feel afterward!

Eat Probiotics!

If you decide to detox it might seem like the list of prohibited foods is huge. However, there are still many great choices for a detox diet and you should still find that you can eat a diverse and tasty diet during your detox and body cleanse.

In particular, PROBIOTICS are a good choice. Probiotics are a group of foods that contain 'good' bacteria that promote a healthy gastrointestinal ecosystem. As you may know, your gut contains tens of thousands of different bacteria, some of which can benefit your health, some which cause harm and some which have little impact. The health of the bowels is increasingly understood to be crucial to human health, with some studies suggesting that the flora of the gut influencing how many nutrients and calories you absorb from your food and even contributing to mood swings and depressions. In fact, probiotics have also been argued to help prevent diarrhea, gut disease, and improve eczema although the support for these claims is controversial.

There are many different probiotic foods, including yogurt, sauerkraut, miso soup, kefir, sourdough bread and tempeh, all of which are considered healthy detox-friendly foods, at least when eaten in moderation. Probiotics can also be found as a supplement, although if you decide to take a specific probiotic supplement it's worth further researching what the proposed benefits are – there are many different types of probiotic supplement all of the different supposed effects.

Changing your Eating Habits

Whether you are attempting a detox diet or trying to fast, you are not only working against your natural instinct to eat but any habits and emotions that revolve around food. You might eat when you are tired to give you a boost in energy, binge to perk up your mood or make poor choices just out of routine or mindlessness. Regardless of your reasons for a detox diet or a fast to work, you need to control how you interact with food.

Start by thinking about your current habits. Are you an emotional eater? Do you like to reward yourself with food? The first stage to overcoming these habits is simply recognizing them and being honest with yourself. It's better to admit your faults rather than to pretend that they don't exist; they'll be there regardless.

By acknowledging how you interact with food you can anticipate and prepare for any temptations that occur during your fast or detox. By depriving yourself of food or by forcing yourself to eat a cleansing diet, you will encounter these feelings and they will probably be stronger than they usually are.

Learn to challenge your feelings and your thoughts. Are you really hungry? Do you really need to give up on your fast? Isn't there alternate, more productive way to deal with your emotions? Try meditating or doing some active, such as walking your dog or tackling a task you've been putting off. By engaging with an activity you consider positive you'll feel much better afterward and the emotions that were bothering you will dissipate.

Also, learn to just sit and be comfortable with your feelings. Instead of shying away from the emotional pain that might be driving you to binge eat, or simply the lack of motivation to continue, take a moment to pause in your day and explore these feelings. Are they strong or weak? How do they affect your thought patterns? How are these feelings affecting your body – can you explore where these feelings are actually occurring? The more you learn to delve into these feelings instead of running away, the more mundane they will become and the less influence they will have over you.

You should also make an effort to be mindful of your eating patterns, in both a detox diet and an eating pattern that involves fasting. You might find that you gorge on your food without truly considering or tasting it, or when you come home from work you automatically start browsing around in the fridge for something to snack on. By trying to be more aware of your interactions with food, you can help manage temptations and habits that urge you to eat.

Finally, try to think positively about your detox diet or fast. Studies have shown that it's easier to change your habits by developing positive habits, rather than breaking negative habits. Or in other words, instead of thinking 'I want to stop feeling so lethargic and bloating it's better to think 'I want to be successful in my detox diet'. These two thoughts might relate to the same goal, but the latter has a much more positive vibe to it, which also makes it easier to strive towards.

Dealing with Other People

Many people won't appreciate the benefits of fasting or a detox diet. You can cite a hundred different studies or try to explain your motivations as logically and clearly as possible, but people might still sneer or disregard what you are doing.

As a result, it's best to consider carefully who you talk about your diet. Do they need to know? Does it bother you if you don't have their approval? It might not be a big deal if someone doesn't accept your diet, but it can still make your life easier if you are not listening to snide comments or objections every time you are around them.

You can always find support online or a detox and fasting community nearby to talk to. These people will understand you and be more welcoming. Of course, you may be fortunate to be surrounded by friends and family who are considerate, or at the very least, appreciate what you are doing is important to you.

If you have to tell people, just try and be as clear and reasonable about the discussion as possible. Laying a strong foundation for why you are doing a fast or detox diet will help people accept it; if your first explanation is watertight, people will find it hard to object, yet if you explain yourself poorly, you'll be dogged by criticism throughout.

Chapter 9: Keto Diet And Autophagy

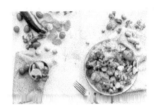

If intermittent fasting has been a trend over the last few years, then the keto diet is its sister. A lot of people have realized the benefits that accrue due to following the two modes of eating and incorporate them hand in hand to fully realize their benefits. To understand the essence of the keto diet and how it induces autophagy, we shall first delve into the basics.

A keto diet is simply a meal plan which involves restricting the amount of carbohydrates taken into the body through total elimination or restricting the consumption to very low amounts in every meal. To understand the shift of eating that is the keto diet, it is imperative to learn about the general functionality of the body.

The body needs energy for all of its functions. From simple activities such as breathing to vital activities such as maintaining a constant heartbeat and brain function, there must be energy. The primary source of energy in the body is glucose, which is obtained after the consumption of carbohydrates. When one ingests the carbs, they are broken down into simple sugars and the energy obtained is used as fuel for the body's functions. There are two body hormones which control the level of glucose and consequent energy obtained from the carbohydrates. The hormones are insulin and glucagon.

When you ingest carbohydrates, the immediate effect is a spike in the level of blood glucose which sends a signal to the pancreas to release the regulatory hormone insulin. Insulin helps facilitate the absorption of sugars from the bloodstream and into the body's cells where they are used as a source of energy. Depending on the amount of carbohydrates consumed, there is a high chance that excessive carbohydrates will not be completely used up. On the contrary, the cells use up the energy needed and the rest is stored as glycogen in the liver and the muscle cells.

As more glucose is transferred from the bloodstream to the cells, the overall level of blood glucose drops. It results in reduced insulin production, and accompanying release of the hormone glucagon. Typically, glucagon is released around four hours after a meal, assuming that you do not ingest any other carbohydrates. The glucagon prompts the conversion of stored glycogen into glucose, which is then released into the bloodstream and used up as energy by other cells.

Assuming that a person keeps eating foods high in carbohydrates, it is a fact that the insulin hormone would be at work more than glucagon. And the result is increased conversion of the excess glucose into glycogen. In simple terms, the result is consistent weight gain.

The keto diet aims at reducing the amount of carbohydrates consumed, the result of which is the decline of insulin production and the activation of the glucagon hormone. When the body is deprived of carbs, glucagon is produced and it helps in the release of glucose stored in the liver and muscle cells back into the bloodstream for use by the other cells. As is evident, the more the glucose released, the more weight loss and control of terminal ailments

The whole essence of following a keto diet is achieving a state known as Ketosis. Ketosis is a metabolic state which shifts the source of energy from glucose to compounds known as ketones. As previously discussed, the body obtains its energy through the glycolysis process when one ingests carbohydrates. Since the food you consume is stored in the form of glucose to a larger extent, then fats and proteins, ketosis aims at activating the source of energy to shift from glucose to fats and proteins. The only way through which this situation can be achieved is by first eliminating the glycogen stores. The only way through which they can be eliminated is through the avoidance of more storage and ensuring that the available stores are converted and used up by the body. Since the glucose is obtained from carbs, it is obvious that they need to be cut down significantly (5% of the entire diet), to activate ketosis.

Once the glycogen stores are depleted, the body begins converting fat stored in the body into simple compounds known as ketones. Just like glucose, the ketones now become the key molecule providing the body with sufficient energy, which shifts the metabolism from reliance on carbs to eating itself. When ketosis occurs, the rate of burn of the fat therein is extremely high. And most keto dieters realize very fast weight loss as one of the initial signs of the effectiveness of the diet.

Usually, the conversion of the fat into ketones takes place in the liver. Once done, the ketones then enter the bloodstream and are used as sources of fuel by the cells throughout the body. Entering ketosis may be very difficult at the beginning, since indulging in anything that would trigger glycolysis automatically puts one out of the keto state. Therefore, if you have made up your mind to practice the keto diet, you must be committed to the diet in entirety and avoid any instance where glycolysis may be triggered. If the latter occurs, you have to take as much time as you did during the first time to achieve ketosis again.

How to Achieve Ketosis

As discussed, the body only enters ketosis when it shifts entirely from reliance on glucose to a reliance on ketones for energy. Once you achieve ketosis, you immediately get to autophagy. There are several ways to enter the ketosis state easily:

1. Elimination/Limitation of the Consumption of Carbs

As has been discussed, the first step toward achieving ketosis is following a diet that is so low in carbs to the point that the body cannot rely on the food consumed to produce energy. When the glycogen stores are depleted, the body has no option but to shift to ketosis where the stored fats are broken down into ketones.

Notably, the level to which carbohydrates must be minimized is not the same for everyone and, in fact, varies drastically amongst different people. A large proportion of people have to take less than 20g of carbs at any given day while people with a high metabolism can eat a slightly higher number of carbs and still achieve ketosis. In the current time, there are hundreds of online apps which help in the calculation of both calories and carb contents. You can use them in the case you are not sure about the composition.

You must be wary of some vegetables. Although vegetables are often thought to be healthy, some have very high carb content and would disrupt you from achieving ketosis. Opponents of the diet assert that it is too complicated and that it takes a lot of time and money to follow. However, the truth is that the meal plan is quite simple, and people can work with what they have and achieve ketosis in the long run. Aim at eating protein and fatty foods in higher amounts than carbs.

2. **Increasing your rate of physical activity**

When you are aiming at achieving ketosis, what you are usually aiming for is to reduce the glycogen stores as fast as possible so that the body can shift to the use of ketones. Physical activities increase the energy requirements in the body, which causes the glycogen stores to be broken down faster and allows you to achieve ketosis. Studies show that when you exercise, you have a 314% chance of achieving ketosis more quickly.

3. Consumption of coconut oil and healthy fats

Coconut oil is one of the foods which have high levels of medium-chain triglycerides (MCT's). These oils are very rare and have the major advantage of being easily absorbed into the body. Once absorbed, they are directly taken to the liver and used up as a major source of the energy needed to convert body fat into ketones. The level of oil consumed is directly related to the number of ketones in the body. Therefore, aim to consume as much of these oils as possible.

Healthy fats are also a major component of the ketogenic diet. Since the fats contain calories, they should amount to 70-80% of the total caloric intake. The shift and transition from a normal diet to a fatty diet is often a bit difficult at the beginning since the body is not accustomed to the digestion of such high fat content foods. Some of the healthy fats advised in the quest to achieve ketosis include:

• Oils from fatty meats such as eggs and ghee

• Plant-based fats such as avocado and olive oil

• Natural fats such as coconut and virgin olive oil

4. *Hydration*

Water is one of the most important digestion components as well as an enabler of the elimination of body toxins. In addition to the benefits, water also enables the transportation of nutrients throughout the body as it is well known that water is the major compound in blood.

It explains why it has such a pivotal role in the transportation of nutrients. In addition to the transportation capabilities, water helps the liver to metabolize fats during ketosis.

It is also well known that dehydration significantly affects the kidneys. Since the kidneys are responsible for the elimination of waste, poor hydration causes a buildup of toxins and a subsequent poor elimination of the same. The result is a disruption of the body's normal processes and, in particular, the inhibition of the burning of body fat. Such an occurrence results in a slow ketosis process. Further, dehydration also affects liver function and the result is a failure to produce sufficient ketone bodies.

It is worth noting that the keto diet is in itself very dehydrating. The ketosis process is very different from the glycolysis process. In the latter, glucose is broken down into energy and water, which helps in body hydration. Ketones do not release any water molecules when they're utilized. It is the major cause of excessive dehydration. Therefore, you should drink plenty of water as often as possible.

5. *Fasting*

Fasting is undoubtedly one of the fastest ways to achieve ketosis. As discussed in chapter 2, there are many ways through which you can fast. The most common fasting strategy is intermittent fasting where one follows a strategy that defines the eating window and the duration where one should be fasting. Fasting is not easy and requires the utmost commitment and dedication. However, it remains to be the best approach to achieve ketosis more quickly. You should identify the plan which works for you and adopt it.

6. Eating more protein

Proteins are key ingredients in the keto diet. As has been described, the body may resolve to break down the body's fats and proteins when there is no longer any glucose available from carbohydrates. If you do not consume enough protein, the body uses up the muscular protein and it may not always be appealing. Always aim to ensure that each of the meals consumed has some protein to prevent the digestion of your muscles.

How Ketosis Boosts Autophagy

The essence of ketosis in itself boosts autophagy through the elimination of carbs and subsequent ensuring that the body uses up body fat and proteins as a source of energy. As described, calorie restriction is the fastest way of achieving autophagy. However, calorie restriction is not the only way through which the keto diet manages to induce and maintain autophagy. Other benefits that accrue include:

1. Mitochondrial biogenesis. *The mitochondria are responsible for the transportation of energy within the cells, hence are referred to as the powerhouse of the cells. These organelles help in the production of over 90% of the body's energy needs through a process known as oxidative phosphorylation. The process involves the combination of oxygen with vital micronutrients obtained through the keto diet, to create the cellular energy known as ATP. Without proper nutrition, the production of ATP is inhibited and the result is an increase of free radicals in the body, known as oxidative stress. Through mitochondrial biogenesis, new and healthy cells are developed, and the damaged cells are replaced. This is basically the whole concept of autophagy, where cell regeneration takes place.*

2. Improved insulin signaling. *Insulin helps in the regulation of blood glucose whenever one eats foods that have a high carb or sugar content. Some times, the body may stop responding to the blood glucose levels, either due to constant spiking of blood glucose which causes the liver to wear out or due to some genetic predisposition. When the body stops responding to the sugars, insulin resistance is said to ensue. The keto diet helps reverse any instance of insulin resistance through the lowering of the overall blood glucose levels as a result of a low carb diet. It gives the liver time to redevelop, and the ultimate result is an increase in insulin response. It is known as increased insulin signaling.*

Maintaining Ketosis

If achieving ketosis is hard, then maintaining it is even more difficult. Once you embark on the ketogenic journey, there is an immense need to ensure that you remain in ketosis until you achieve your dietary and weight goals. The only way through which you can ensure that you remain in ketosis is by ensuring that no glycolysis takes place and that the body runs purely on ketones. It is worth understanding that a simple mistake in the meal plan can take a person out of ketosis and that this could be as simple as eating a small sugary meal. Carbohydrate intake must be kept at the minimum if the ketosis state is to be maintained.

In the case you are having difficulty with some of the elements of the diet, cyclic ketogenic dieting may be the best option for you. The strategy involves sticking to a strict keto diet for an extended period and then taking a day or two off and eating normally. The major benefit of this strategy is that it helps curb cravings since you will be able to indulge in the foods that you want during this "off" period. The freedom and satisfaction of the cravings ensure that you are mentally prepared for the next phase of dieting. This period is normally referred to as the "cheat window", and it gives the body a break from using ketones as the primary source of energy.

As we have discussed, autophagy is, in most instances, activated by energy deprivation. To achieve energy deprivation, one or more of the following conditions must hold:

● There must be an amino acid deficiency.

● There must be glucose restriction.

● You must be fasting.

● You need low insulin levels in the blood.

On the other hand, ketosis is achieved when the body is under glucose restriction. With this realization, it is evident that achieving ketosis undoubtedly helps achieve autophagy. The more the ketosis process proceeds, the higher the rate of autophagy.

It is a fact that ketosis mimics fasting. When you are in the fasting mode, the body does not have glucose to help in the production of energy but relies on the breakdown of protein into ketones which are used as the source of the required energy. In ketosis, the body relies on ketones too. Ultimately, autophagy is achieved just as easily during the diet as it is when a person is fasting for real.

As is evident, being in a ketosis state meets most of the prerequisites of autophagy, including low insulin levels and low blood glucose. The basis is always the amount of glucose you are taking into the body. When you keep up with a strict keto diet, your insulin levels remain low and autophagy begins thereafter. Keeping up with the keto diet ensures that autophagy continues for a long period, and you get to enjoy the benefits for a longer duration.

The most natural method of achieving autophagy while on the keto diet is to ensure that you do not do anything which will get you out of ketosis for a long period. When ketosis is prolonged, you can be sure that the stored glycogen has been depleted and that ketone production is ramped up.

When it comes to amino acid deficiency, it is important to note that ketosis promotes a form of autophagy known as macro-autophagy. While you are in the ketosis state, the body has a high chance of recycling particular proteins through a process known as chaperone-mediated autophagy. To achieve this, you have to make sure that you are not eating too much protein since it results in the build-up of amino acids. Also, you have to ensure that you are quite strategic when it comes to the determination of your eating window, and you can link up the keto diet with intermittent fasting. That means that, unlike the normal IF strategy where you are allowed to eat whatever you want, you can opt to only indulge in keto-friendly meals during your eating window.

Chapter 10: Activating Autophagy Through Fasting

Experts say that fasting is the fastest and most effective way to help the body to get into a state of autophagy[53]. How does that happen? Fasting deprives the body of nutrients which signals the body to activate autophagy. When we stop eating the body's insulin levels go down. And to compensate for that drop in insulin drop, the body produces more glucagon. When you have more glucagon it triggers autophagy[54].

Researchers like the award winning Yoshinori Ohsumi and plenty of others recommend fasting (particularly intermittent fasting) as a means to activating autophagy. There are other methods of course, such as the Ketogenic diet for instance, but we will go over those in a separate chapter. In this chapter we will focus on fasting and how you can use it to induce autophagy.

What is Fasting?

Isn't fasting the equivalent of starvation? Well, not exactly—but yes you will starve at one point. The big difference between general starvation and the practice of fasting is control. Starvation is involuntary—you are forced to it due to the lack of food. On the other hand fasting is not—you chose not to eat.

Starvation can lead to severe health problems and even death. Fasting on the other hand is controlled and deliberate and you can stop any time you want. Yes, you will suffer from the lack of food in both cases but you as you can see you have control when you fast.

Fasting for Religious and Spiritual Purposes

People have been fasting for a lot of different reasons for thousands of years now. Some do it for health reasons while others do it for spiritual reasons. Yes, spiritual reasons.

For instance, Muslims go fasting during the month of Ramadan—they fast for an entire month. Catholics on the other hand do fasting every Good Friday and on Ash Wednesday. On Yom Kippur, Jews undergo a six day fast.

Hindus on the other hand have several new moon fasts like the Shivarati, Saraswati, and Puja. Mormons go fasting on the first Sunday of every month. Other religious traditions that include fasting are those from Jainists, Taoists, and Buddhists.

Fasting for Health and Fitness

Fasting as a practice has been around for thousands of years. So, it's not really new. But you don't have to be religious to go on a fast. Fasting is also a practice for people who are not underweight. Some people try fasting to lose weight. Note however, that if you have health issues you should consult with your doctor first before trying any form of fasting.

Bodybuilders in particular have been looking to cut down on body fat through fasting. You see, when the food supply is cut, the body will start to use its stored energy to survive—the stored body fat to be exact.

During fasting you choose not to eat for health reasons—maybe to cut weight, stimulate autophagy for healing, and other reasons. Food is readily available. You will also have a designated fasting period. After the fasting period you will have to eat and thus end your fast.

Some undergo fasting for a day up to several days with medical supervision. Sometimes you will be required by your doctor to fast before undergoing a medical procedure. But that is a different subject altogether.

You may not know it but you actually undergo fasting every night. You've been doing it your entire life. Do you know where the word "breakfast" comes from and what it means?

Break-Fast

This term actually comes from "break fast"—it is the meal that people eat to break their fasting period. You eat breakfast in the morning; that means you were actually fasting as you slept at night. That implicitly means we all fast at night and it is something that we do daily.

However this nightly fast is actually a short term fast usually lasting anywhere from 6 to 10 hours. Some people sleep longer for various reasons. Body builders and people who are sick need to sleep in order to recuperate.

Benefits of Fasting
- **Weight Loss** – as stated earlier there are people who undergo fasting to lose

weight. Any extra that gets digested and doesn't get used by the body will end up getting stored for later use. That stored unused body fuel is called fat. Since fasting means not eating the body will switch to using fat for sustenance.

- **Promotes Longevity** – as you grow older your metabolism slows down. This condition will later lead to a gradual loss of muscle tissue, which is known as sarcopenia. The good news is that fasting helps to speed up your metabolism, which prevents sarcopenia and the degradation of muscular tissue. On top of that fasting triggers autophagy.
- **Detoxifies the Body** – nutrient deprivation is interpreted by the brain as a form of stress or threat and it reacts protectively or defensively. The brain starts up its adaptive stress response and that includes looking for

alternative sources of energy. The liver is then triggered to produce glycogen as an alternative source. After that the body turns to fat stores—when that happens the toxins in the fat get released in the conversion process when fat is used as an energy source.

- **Metabolic Boost** – as it was explained earlier, the body gets a metabolic boost when you go fasting. According to one study[55], fasting can boost the body's metabolism by up to 14%. According to another medical study, people who undergo fasting experience an increase in neropinephrine in their blood. This is a neurotransmitter that increases the body's metabolism.

Improves Brain Function – studies suggest that undergoing fasting may help to improve overall brain function. It promotes the production of BNDF or brain-derived neurotrophic factor. BNDF helps protect the brain from degenerative conditions such as Alzheimer's and Parkinson's disease. According to one study, it is suggested that fasting helps to improve memory[56]—this is according to the Society for Neuroscience. Another study suggests that fasting also promotes the growth of new nerve cells[57].

In the next chapter we will go over what intermittent fasting is and its various forms.

Chapter 11: Autophagy As A Regulator Of Body Weight

Some people suggest that eating only one meal per day can improve your health and thus, supporting the concept of intermittent fasting. Though there is not much evidence, that supports that intermittent fasting actually helps to improve autophagy, there is a plethora of knowledge that exercise is quite beneficial to the process.

Using autophagy fasting for weight loss

Let's go by the idea that intermittent fasting helps with autophagy, it also then means that it will help in your weight loss journey as well. All you need to do is make the necessary changes to your lifestyle dieting, exercise, sleep, etc., that will allow you to support it. So, as you fine-tune your diet, you are able to use the process of autophagy to help you lose those extra pounds, as it makes your metabolic processes more efficient.

Autophagy, fat burning and a healthier body

Scientists have recognized that the key to slow down the aging process is through autophagy. You can do so by restricting the amount of protein you eat for an entire day. This is called a protein fast. On this diet, you will provide your bodies with benefits such as weight loss and anti-aging benefits. When you consume less protein in a day (less than 15 grams) then your body will look for other ways to recycle proteins.

This also means that your insulin levels will be low, and your body will not store the fat from food ingested. Further research is being done so that it can be known how autophagy can be targeted in the cells to help cure and diminish the debilitating effects of Parkinson's disease, Type 2 diabetes and cancer.

So, what are the best methods for managing weight and staying in shape?

Fasting has become a popular weight loss trend over the last few years, because it helps us to control more effectively the number of calories we consume. It is also beneficial because it promotes the process of autophagy and helps to protect us from diseases. The different types of fasting are known as intermittent fasting.

They are adaptable and you are allowed to determine the times in which you eat the normal amount of calories, your body requires and also the times in which you do not eat. At the times you do not eat, you may eat a few calories, or you may have no calories at all.

Research shows that intermittent fasting, reduces the overall fat in our bodies and findings suggest that it improves or cardio-metabolic. Even though this is seen in studies that are conducted with mice where it shows that they live longer. These findings are used to conclude how these will help us as well and will propel further research in the field. So, we still have a way to go in understanding the relationship between intermittent fasting and our overall health.

However, what these studies show is that the process of autophagy is a natural occurrence in our bodies and fasting aids in its efficiency. Overall, we have an increased resistance to diseases such as diabetes and obesity and it allows us to live longer and healthier lives.

Chapter 12: Water Fasting For Weight Loss

When we engage in fasting the body lose weight, one of the way we can engage in fasting is by the use of water. When we use water to fast for some days the body will begin to lose weight. Fasting with water for about 5 days, from day two the weight the body will lose is water weight, then from day 3 the weight the body will begin to lose Is fat.

When we don't eat for days the body will convert the fat that have been stored by the body into food for the body, as the body begin to convert fat to food we begin to lose weight. If you want to engage in water fasting, it is good for you to plan before you start water fasting. Planning is very important so that you will not cause damage to your body.

Water Fasting is divided Into 3 phase, which are pre fasting, fasting and post fasting. When you say pre fasting, this has to deal with stage before fasting. In this stage you should prepare the body before you enter the fast. Preparing the body means taking food that is less solid so that the body will begin to understand. In pre fasting stage ensure to take foods that are less solid.

In the fasting stage begin to take water depending on the goal you have set in your mind. Then for the post fasting ensures you do not hurry to break the fast by taking solid food because this can greatly affect the body. When you engage in water fasting ensure to plan properly so that you will not harm your body. Also ensure to work with your doctor so that your doctor can set date suitable for you.

CONCLUSION

So intermittent fasting is available to anyone that is looking for its benefits. If you want to lose weight, balance insulin levels, age slower, get rid of brain fog, support detoxification, then the intermittent fasting is great for you. Bear in mind that intermittent fasting is not for pregnant women. Of course, it's not that complicated to do, but its better that you avoid fasting during your copulation period. If you have diabetes, then try working with a portioned to make sure that you are eating the right foods. If you have diabetes, then intermittent fasting will help to cure diabetes, if you eat a diet containing fiber, fats, and protein without any sugar and carbs.

Ideally, with intermittent fasting, it is advisable to start eating your first meal of the day around noon or 1pm, and then eat your last meal around 5 or 6 pm...and then skip meals for the remaining part of the day until it's about 1pm the next day. Now during the intermittent fasting, you can take a lot of fluids. Remember that when you are doing the intermittent fasting, you need to eat a diet that has lots of nutrients in it. Also, try eating some herbs with whatever diet you are eating. If you are preparing chicken, then throw the herbs into the chicken that you are going to eat. If you are making an Italian chicken dish, then add lots of basil and rosemary to it. If you are making a smoothie, add a teaspoon of sesame in there.

To wrap everything up, there is nothing complex about the intermittent fasting. You are only eating less during the day, and it is very simple to follow. For the first three days, you will have so many cravings, but after a few days, you will no longer be hungry in the morning. You will feel okay until lunchtime. So make sure that you try out the intermittent fasting tomorrow!